EPIDEMIOLOGY

Epidemiology

Published by Quantum Scientific Publishing a division of Sentient Enterprises, Inc. Pittsburgh, PA. Copyright © 2017 by Sentient Enterprises, Inc. All rights reserved.

Permission in writing must be obtained from the publisher before any part of this work may be reproduced or transmitted in any form or by any means, electronic or mechanical, including photocopying and recording, or by any information storage or retrieval system. All trademarks, service marks, registered trademarks, and registered service marks are the property of their respective owners and are used herein for identification purposes only.

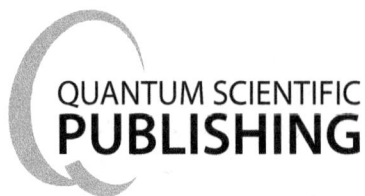

table of CONTENTS

Chapter 1 – Introduction to Epidemiology 1

Chapter 2 – John Snow's Story of Cholera 5

Chapter 3 – Infectious Epidemiology 9

Chapter 4 – Environmental Epidemiology 15

Chapter 5 – Psychosocial Epidemiology 21

Chapter 6 – Forensic Epidemiology 25

Chapter 7 – Ecological Study Design 31

Chapter 8 – Cross-sectional Study Design 37

Chapter 9 – Case-control Study Design 43

Chapter 10 – Cohort Study Design 47

Chapter 11 – Randomized Controlled Trial (RCT) Study Design 51

Chapter 12 – Surveillance and Mortality Data 55

Chapter 13 – Screening 61

Chapter 14 – Prevalence and Incidence 67

Chapter 15 – Ethics 71

Chapter 16 – Risk Factors 77

Chapter 17 – Sample, Population, and Sample Size 81

Chapter 18 – Sources of Data 85

Chapter 19 – Types of Surveys and Variables 89

Chapter 20 – Constructing Survey Questions 93

Chapter 21 – Answer Choices and Layout in Survey Construction 99

Chapter 22 – Survey Layout 103

Chapter 23 – Use of Incentives and Participation Proportion 107

Chapter 24 – Biomarker Matrices and Collection 111

Chapter 25 – Making a Map – MAUP 119

Chapter 26 – Chloropleth Maps 123

Chapter 27 – Making a Map – Elements 129

Chapter 28 – Use of Tables in Reporting Results 133

Chapter 29 – Graphs and Charts 137

Chapter 30 – Person, Time, and Place 143

Chapter 31 – Causality 147

Chapter 32 – Sampling Error and Chance 157

Chapter 33 – Sampling Frame 161

Chapter 34 – Confounding and Effect Modifier 165

Chapter 35 – Types of Bias 173

Chapter 36 – Generalizability 177

Chapter 37 – Publication Bias 181

Chapter 38 – Crude Rate, Numerator and Denominator 185

Chapter 39 – Direct Standardization 191

Chapter 40 – Indirect Standardization 195

Chapter 41 – Relative Risk 199

Chapter 42 – Odds Ratio 203

Chapter 43 – Confidence Interval 207

Chapter 44 – Evidence-Based Research 211

Chapter 45 – Public Policy 215

Chapter 1 - Introduction to Epidemiology

Chapter Objectives

- Define epidemiology
- Describe what epidemiologists do
- List where epidemiologists work

What is Epidemiology?

The most common guess is that it is a skin disease. You probably remember from biology that the outermost layer of the skin is called the epidermis. From Greek and Latin roots, "epi" means "outside" and "derm" means skin. Therefore, epidermis means outside layer of skin. However, epidemiology is not a skin disease.

Three Greek words make up the term, epidemiology: "epi" means on or upon; "demos" means people; and "logos" means the study of. Therefore, epi demi ology means the study of what is upon the people.

The formal definition of epidemiology is the study of the distribution and determinants of health related states in specific populations, and the application of this controlled study of health problems.

In more basic terms, it is the study of diseases in populations.

Epidemiology looks at epidemics (sudden increase) and endemic (always present) diseases. One of the underlying beliefs of epidemiologists is that disease does not occur at random. In other words, epidemiologists believe that there is some pattern to the disease. It may be related to the persons, place or time.

What do Epidemiologists do?

Epidemiologists are disease detectives. They work with others to figure out the reason for health problems in a community, region, country or countries.

They use special tools to look for clues. They count the number of people who have a disease or injury in a community, region, country, or countries. Using math, they figure out if there is a pattern of disease or if a problem exists.

Just like police detectives, they gather information in a systematic way. Systematic means getting things done using clearly defined steps. As in other scientific disciplines, epidemiology uses the scientific method to define questions, design and perform the experiment, and analyze and present the data.

When epidemiologists solve the problem or have a good idea about why the problem occurred, they let the public know. This can happen in many ways, such as making announcements through the media, suggesting a change in a law, and educating the public.

Epidemiologists also use their understanding to prevent further illness or disease. They do this by making suggestions about what factors may play a role in the pattern of disease or illness. An example is health inspectors for restaurants making sure the pork is cooked enough because we know pork that is not thoroughly cooked may cause illness.

Where do Epidemiologists Work?

Epidemiologists work in many different places. Some epidemiologists work in the local health department. In the health department, one job of an epidemiologist may be to figure out the reason for an outbreak of food poisoning or whether a neighborhood has more children in that neighborhood diagnosed with childhood leukemia than in other neighborhoods. Some epidemiologists work in hospitals, non-profit organizations, or in large governmental agencies, such as Centers for Disease Control and Prevention (CDC) or the World Health Organization (WHO). Epidemiologists in these larger governmental agencies often work on health issues at the national or international level. For example, CDC and WHO would be involved in understanding the spread of avian influenza or any cases of poliomyelitis (short name is polio). Another group of epidemiologist works in universities. These epidemiologists either work on describing the whos, whats, whens, and wheres of a disease or the whys and hows of a disease. In other words, they do the research that uncovers relationships between different factors and disease. This information is used to help improve the health of populations by establishing health programs and policies.

What have Epidemiologists Taught Us?

Many truths about disease and illness were discovered by epidemiologists. A hundred and fifty years ago (mid 1850s), an epidemiologist showed that cholera was spread through contaminated water. Remember, this was *before* we knew about bacteria. About 50 years ago, epidemiologists (the Framingham Study, started in 1948) were able to tell us about risk factors for heart attacks and strokes. Before then, we had little knowledge about who was at risk for a heart attack or stroke or why some people were more likely to have a heart attack or stroke and others were not. Epidemiologists were the first to show that cigarette smoking was linked to lung cancer (Drs. Doll and Hill; study in the mid 1950s). Epidemiologists were also important is showing that a drug given to pregnant women, diethylstilbestrol (DES), harmed their babies. However, this harm did not occur until the children reached adolescence or young adulthood. One of the harms was that daughters of mothers who took DES could develop a rare cancer of the vagina or cervix. Epidemiologists have taught us a lot about the health of people.

Summary

Epidemiology is the study of health and disease in populations. Epidemiologists are interested in both epidemic and endemic diseases. Epidemics are sudden increases in the incidence of a disease. Endemic diseases are those that exist at a stable level in a population. Epidemiologists work to figure out the causes of diseases in specific areas or populations. They use the knowledge they gain to prevent future disease. Many of the laws about restaurants and sanitation are based on epidemiological research. Public health inspectors have the job of enforcing those laws to help prevent outbreaks of disease. Epidemiologists have also helped us understand the way disease spreads through a population.

Concept Reinforcement

1. Explain epidemiology and discuss what epidemiologists do.

2. Explain why epidemiologists work in so many different types of organizations.

3. Discuss the role of epidemiologists played in understanding the effects of DES.

Chapter 2 - John Snow's Story of Cholera

Chapter Objectives

- Describe John Snow's cholera story
- List the important finding of Snow's study
- Describe the two competing beliefs about health at that time

Around two hundred years ago, death spread from India, China, Russia, Western Europe and then to North America. The reason was cholera. It is an infectious disease caused by a bacteria. Millions of people died of cholera. It was one of the most rapidly fatal diseases known. A person could die within 3 hours of falling sick. At that time, it was one of the most feared diseases because it seemed to make people look less human because they seemed to shrink due to loss of water from diarrhea. Although there are still people who get cholera in the world today, it is no longer a disease that kills millions.

Beliefs About Cholera in the Mid-1800s

Bad Air Belief

In London, there were two main schools of thought about the cause of cholera. One group of people believed that cholera was caused by miasma. Miasma means bad air. People try to protect themselves by wearing sweet smelling herbs. Men smoked large cigars. Because of the miasma belief, London officials searched for bad smells. Below is a cartoon showing the search for bad smells.

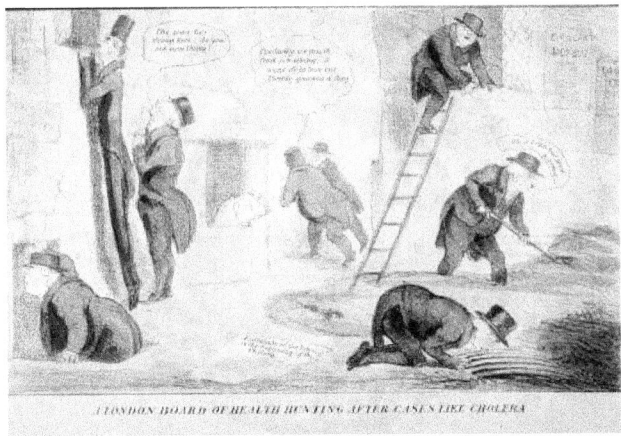

Cartoon showing search for bad air by London officials

Bad Water Belief

When John Snow was 18 years old and in his 4th year as an apprentice to Dr. Hardcastle, a cholera epidemic hit London. Dr. Hardcastle had so many sick patients that he sent John Snow to treat sick coal miners alone. He could do little to help them and many died. He did a lot of thinking about cholera. In his early 30s, he was a successful doctor in London. He thought that cholera was spread through contaminated water.

Two water companies supplied water to London. One company, the Southwark and Vauxhall Water company, got its water from an area of the Thames River known to be polluted with sewage. The other water company, the Lambeth Water Company, pulled its water north of the city where the water was less polluted.

John Snow showed that people who drank water from the Southwark and Vauxhall Water Company were much more likely to get cholera compared to people who drank water from the Lambeth Water Company. In one month, 286 people who drank water supplied from the Southwark and Vauxhall Water Company died of cholera compared to 14 people who drank water supplied by the Lambeth Water Company.

He wrote and spoke about his findings. Unfortunately, he was not believed. He was one of the first to use a survey of people and look at where the disease was occurring to figure out the cause of the disease.

In August of 1853, anther epidemic hit London in an area close to John Snow's home, which was in the west London district of Soho. John Snow mapped out the places where people died of cholera in one area of London. This area, the Soho area of London, had many, many deaths. The people in the Soho area had one thing in common. They used the Broad Street pump's water.

As further evidence of the culprit, John Snow noted that the work house, which is like a prison, had only 5 deaths. The work house was a smelly place. If the miasma idea was correct, then most of the 55 inmates should have died. In reality, the workhouse was a safe place to live. The workhouse had its own deep well and did not use the Broad Street pump's water. Another local place, the brewery, did not have any deaths. Again, it was a very smelly place. Based on the miasma idea, many people who worked in the brewery should have died of cholera, but no one did. Why? The brewery workers were given free beer to drink, so they did not drink the water.

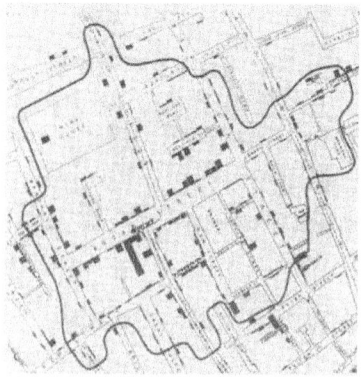

Map made by John Snow showing places that people died in the Soho area of London

After much detective work, John Snow was able to show that the water from one pump, the Broad Street pump, was the source of the disease. However, his idea was not accepted and he died a couple of years later, in 1858, at the age of 45. Finally, in 1884, the bacteria that caused cholera was re-discovered. John Snow's idea was at last believed.

This example of detection work in figuring out the reasons that people get sick or die still continues today. It may be hard to imagine that people had no idea about microscopic organisms and their role in causing sickness and death. Even when John Snow identified the source of cholera as drinking bad water, he did not know what was actually causing the illness. This also is common today in epidemiology—epidemiologists identify the risk factor but not the cause of the disease or death.

Summary

John Snow is known as the father of field epidemiology because he went into the field to gather data. He interviewed people and he mapped the location of cholera deaths to figure out the common factor. In the first stage of John Snow's research into the cause of cholera, he figured out that people who drank the water from Southwark and Vauxhall Water Company were likely to get sick. Next, he went door to door and figured out how many people died of cholera in a small area of London. He also asked them where they got their water. In this area, people usually got their water from the nearest pump, the Broad Street pump. He also found out which water company serviced that pump. Through this detective work, he felt sure that drinking bad water was the reason people got sick and died of cholera. John Snow's efforts to figure out the risk factor for cholera—drinking bad water—, his surveying people to get information about risk factors, and his mapping of the area of cholera deaths, is a classic example of epidemiology.

Concept Reinforcement

1. What factors may have created the situation in which people thought it was bad air that caused the cholera epidemic?(Hint: think about where refuse was deposited in the mid-1800s and rich and poor people's living conditions and nutritional status.)

2. What are two means used in epidemiologic detective work to discover risk factors associated with disease or death?

3. Why would a densely populated city be more susceptible to the cholera epidemic than the rural countryside?

Chapter 3 - Infectious Epidemiology

Chapter Objectives

- State the 3 major factors in infectious disease transmission
- Describe the procedures of investigating an outbreak
- Define herd immunity

Controlling infectious disease is important. Although the United States has fewer deaths these days than 100 years ago from some types of infectious diseases, such as cholera or tuberculosis, some types of infectious diseases still kill many people. For example, pneumonia-influenza was the 8th leading cause of death in 2005 in the Unites States.

Epidemiology Triangle

The epidemiologic triangle is one way to show the major factors necessary for an outbreak.

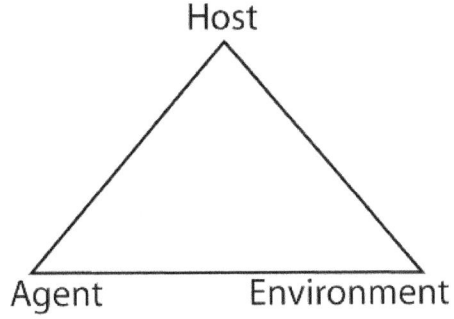

Epidemiology triangle

The Agent

The biological agent in infectious disease is studied in microbiology. In epidemiology, we use the microbiologists' discoveries. For an infection to occur, the agent must be present. There are six types of microbial agents: bacteria, viruses and rickettsia, fungi, protozoa, helminths, and arthropods. Each type of agent causes certain diseases. See the table below for a list.

Agent	Diseases	Comment
Bacteria	TB (Tuberculosis), salmonellosis, streptococcal infections (strep throat)	Leading killers in the 19th century. Antibiotics are used to treat this type of infection. Concern about bacteria resistant to antibiotics.
Viruses and Rickettsia	Hepatitis A, Rocky Mountain Spotted Fever, chicken pox, influenza, AIDS	Virus means poison in Latin. Some people can be carriers of viruses, meaning they do not have any illness but can infect others.
Fungi	Athlete's foot, ringworm	Fungi means mushroom in Latin. Some fungi are used for good, such as yeast to make bread. Others can cause disease.
Protozoa	Malaria, giardiasis, amebiasis	Single cell organisms that cannot be seen with the naked eye. They live in soil, wet sand, and fresh and salt water.
Helminths	Roundworms, tape worms, snail fever	Found in moist tropical regions. Also known as parasitic worms. They live inside the person.
Arthropods	Malaria, Rocky Mountain spotted fever, encephalitis	Living things carry the disease agent: mosquitoes, ticks, flies, mites.

The Environment

The environment means the place where the agent lives. The environment is made up of many factors:

Physical environment

- Humidity
- Weather
- Temperature
- Type of landscape

Social environment of the people

- Culture
- Behavior
- Personality
- Attitudes

For example, in the mid-1800s, water was drawn from the Thames River in London. One water supply company drew its water from the river that was near sewage dumping area. In the warm months of the year, the cholera bacteria could live in this water. Fecal matter (also known as stool or bowel movement) from someone sick with cholera contaminated the water. People who drank this water became sick with cholera. The physical environment consisted of a warm river climate. The social environment consisted of the habit of pouring raw sewage into the local river and drawing drinking water from this river, too.

The Host

An infectious disease agent needs a favorable environment to live. The agent must also have the ability to infect a person. Once infected, a person may or may not show signs of sickness. If the infected person does not get sick, he or she is called a carrier. One very famous carrier was Mary Mallon. She never believed that she infecting people. She felt she was healthy. However, she was a typhoid carrier.

People have ways of blocking infections. Most agents cannot enter our body because our skin protects us. Tears and saliva can wash away infectious agents. Our stomach juice is very acidic and therefore kills many agents. Finally, our immune system can fight infectious agents. However, people still can get an infectious disease.

If a person gets sick, there are four outcomes:

1. Complete recovery. In other words, the person goes back to feeling the same as before the illness.

2. Permanent disability. In this case, the person is not the same as before. For example, if a person gets polio, that person may recover but have a limp. Because the virus destroyed some motor neutrons in the leg, muscle weakness in the leg leads to limping.

3. Disfigurement. A bad break, for example of the pinkie finger, can end up with the pinkie finger not being able to be straightened. This is a disfigurement of the hand.

4. Death. Illness can lead to death.

Typhoid Mary.

Mary Mallon (9/23/1869 – 11/11/1938) was a famous carrier of typhoid. She was a cook for the wealthy in New York City. Health officials discovered that she had infected the families where she was a cook. She was arrested and held in isolation for 3 years at a hospital on North Brother Island. However, Mary Mallon did not feel sick and did not believe that she was a carrier. After 3 years on the island, she agreed to never work as a cook and was freed. However, she started working as a cook again at New York's Sloane Hospital for Women. She infected 25 women there. Mallon was arrested again and sent to the island. She never left the island again.

Herd Immunity

Herd immunity is a term that means that a population, group, or community may not become infected with a disease because most of the people have been vaccinated. In other words, not everyone in a community has to get a vaccine for the whole community to be protected. To become sick with an infectious disease requires contact with another person who has the infection. The likelihood of coming in contact with a infected person is very small when most of a community is vaccinated. For example, if only three-quarters of the population is vaccinated, polio can spread throughout the community. On the other hand, if eighty-five percent of the community is vaccinated, the chance of polio spreading in the community is very low. The exact percent of vaccinated people needed to protect the entire community depends on the disease. For polio, it is approximately 85%. This is called herd immunity. Very few people get polio today in the United States and we do not have epidemics of polio because more than 85% of the children are vaccinated. However, if more and more parents choose to not vaccinate their children against polio, we may see an epidemic because the percent of vaccinated children falls below 85%. So, even if you do not get a vaccine or a flu shot, you can thank those who do get one. They are keeping the community healthy.

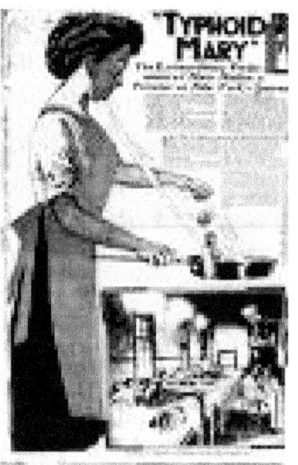

Typhoid Mary

So Who is More Likely to Get an Infectious Disease?

As we grow older, our ability to fight infection decreases. People who do not have balanced diets cannot easily fight infectious diseases. Some people are born with the ability to fight infectious diseases less well than others. It is in their genes. Older people, malnourished people and people born with certain types of genes are more likely to get infectious diseases.

Detecting an Outbreak

An epidemiologist follows five steps in detecting an infectious disease outbreak.

Step 1: Verifying the outbreak

The first step is to make sure there is an outbreak. For example, if a customer in a restaurant said that he became sick because of the food he ate, the epidemiologist would have to make sure he did have food poisoning and not an upset stomach. If there is an outbreak, the emergency room is usually flooded with lots of people with the same complaint. Doctors are very good at making a diagnosis: in this case, whether or not the person had food poisoning.

Step 2: Identification of All People with the Illness

The second step is finding all the people with the disease or illness. Once found, the people describe their symptoms. A laboratory test may also be done at the hospital to help figure out the illness or disease. Mapping where the people were when they began to feel sick also occurs during step 2. Information on the date and time when people felt sick is also gathered. At this point, the epidemiologist may be able to figure out what infectious agent is responsible for the outbreak.

Step 3: Make a Tentative Explanation for the Outbreak

The third step involves making a statement that indicates the possible source of the infection, the likely agent, and the likely method of spread.

Step 4: Compile Evidence

The fourth step involves finding evidence to support or not support the statement made in Step 3. During this time, the search continues for additional infected people.

Step 5: State the Cause of the Outbreak

The fifth and final step uses the results of the investigation to make conclusions. These conclusions may cause a restaurant to close or a beach to shut down. The purpose of the action is to prevent another outbreak.

Summary

No country is immune from infectious diseases, though the important infectious diseases in specific countries vary. One way to fight against some infectious diseases is through vaccination. If most people in a community are vaccinated against an infectious disease, such as polio, it is unlikely that an epidemic will occur. Some diseases cannot be prevented through vaccination and there are outbreaks. If this happens, epidemiologists act as detectives to figure out who was infected and how they were infected. Once this is known, protective action often occurs so others in the community will not become infected.

Concept Reinforcement

1. What do you think about Typhoid Mary? She never felt sick and never believed she was a carrier of Typhoid. Do you agree with her punishment to make her live most of her life on an island?

2. Do you think everyone should be required to get vaccines or is it OK to rely on herd immunity?

3. How are these five steps in investigating an infectious disease outbreak similar to the methods used by police detectives in solving a crime?

Chapter 4 - Environmental Epidemiology

Chapter Objectives

- Define environmental epidemiology
- List the three sources of pollution
- List three factors to consider in exposure to a toxin

In the 21st century, attention has turned to environmental exposures and health outcomes. Some experts believe that about one quarter of the diseases and deaths worldwide are linked to environmental factors. These environmental exposures are outside the control of the exposed individual. These can be from exposure in the workplace, toxic chemicals, indoor and outdoor air pollution.

Albert Einstein, a famous scientist, said "The environment is about everything that is not me." Environmental epidemiologists look at environmental exposures that are related to health. The definition of environmental epidemiology is the study of diseases and illnesses linked to environmental factors. There are many kinds of health problems, such as cancer, birth defects, or infectious diseases. Each one of these may be linked to environmental exposures.

There are three types of sources of pollution:

- Point sources
- Line sources
- Area sources

The type of pollution source plays a role in solving the problem of where the exposure is coming from. If the source can be identified, solutions can be proposed to reduce or eliminate this exposure.

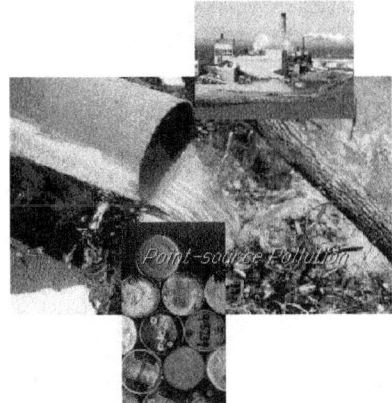

Example of point source pollution

Point source means that the pollution comes from one place. That place can be identified. Factories are point sources. The smokestack or the discharge pipe are both examples of point sources in factories. Containers full of toxins are also a point source. You can point to the place where the exposure begins.

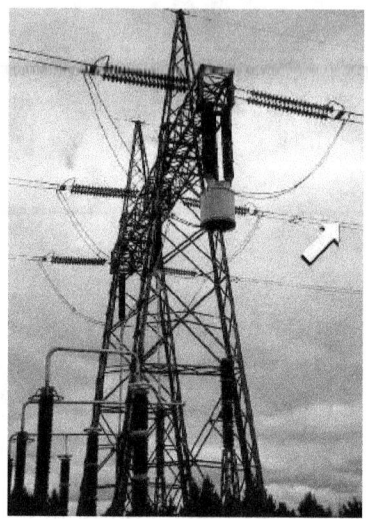

Example of line source pollution: Electrical transmission towers and high-voltage power lines near Albuquerque, New Mexico. The arrow indicates place where crackling sound is heard.

The best example of a line source of pollution is power lines. Another common line source of pollution comes from vehicular exhaust along a highway. Like point sources, line sources can be easily seen. The difference between the two is that point sources are in one place, whereas line sources follow a line of exposure—along the line of high-voltage power lines or along the line of a highway.

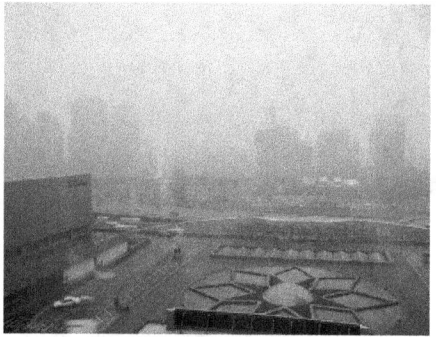

Example of area source pollution: Air pollution in Beijing China

Areas sources of pollution come from afar. The origin may be a line or point source, but the affected area faces pollution of its entire area. Air contaminants from sources far away can create local air pollution problems. Local water can be contaminated by toxins that are carried from point or line sources and fall into the local water. This can contaminate the local water.

There are many examples of mass illness, disease or death linked to environmental exposure over time.

Examples of Environment Exposures Linked to Health

The Great Fog of London

A great fog fell on London in 1952. At first, Londoners did not realize that this fog was a sign of disaster. They were used to fog. However, many things came together to make this fog deadly. When it finally lifted, about 12,000 people died, mostly from breathing problems. This was one of the first disasters that made people realize that the quality of the air is strongly linked to health. This is an example of area source of exposure, the air pollution.

These days, it is common to hear about ozone alert days in the summer. These are days in which ozone, an air pollutant, is high and people who have trouble breathing need to be careful.

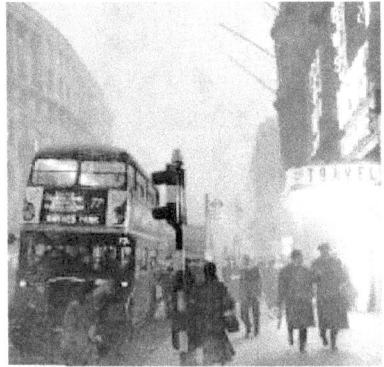

Great fog of London in 1952

Love Canal

Hooker Chemical Company made a canal and filled it with hazardous chemicals, topped the canal with dirt, and sold it to the city of Love Canal for $1. In the late 1950s, about 100 homes and a school were built on this land. Many of the homeowners did not realize they were living on top of a toxic waste dump. Through natural weathering, the buried toxic waste containers migrated to the surface and leaked their contents. Children playing returned home with burns on their hands and faces from these chemicals.

One of the health effects from exposure to these toxic chemicals was birth defects and childhood cancer. In 1978, President Carter approved emergency financial aid to help deal with Love Canal. The State of New York bought the homes of 221 residents so they could move somewhere else. This is an example of point source of exposure–the containers filled with toxins.

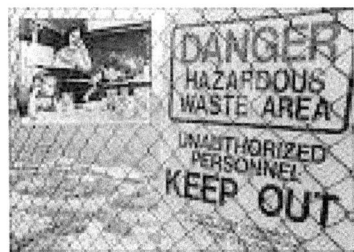

Love Canal, New York

Times Beach

A dusty small town outside of St. Louis Missouri hired Russell Bliss, a waste hauler, to oil the roads in the town. He sprayed the roads with his oil mixture from 1972-1976. Unknown to the residents of Times Beach, the oil was not just used oil but it had large amount of other toxins, including dioxin. Dioxin is thought to be the most toxic chemical made by man. After flooding in 1982, the Environmental Protection Agency (EPA) found dangerous levels of dioxin in Times Beach's soil. The federal government bought the homes of Times Beach residents and evacuated the town in 1983. The former residents of Times Beach were shunned by people in their new communities. People were afraid that exposure to dioxin was contagious (which it is not). Over 265,000 tons of soil were collected and burned from March 1996 to June 1997 to get rid of the dioxin. The cleanup cost was $110 million dollars. This is an example of an exposure beginning at a line source–the oiled roads.

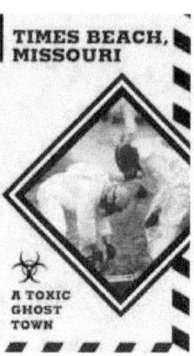

Times Beach, Missouri

Gulf War Syndrome

In the previous examples, the link between environmental exposure and health outcomes has been determined. In case of Gulf War syndrome, much is unknown.

By the late 1990s about 15% of the 700,000 US veterans of the Gulf War complained of health problems. The combat vets say that their health problems are linked to something that happened to them while serving in the war. Some of the wide-ranging symptoms are chronic fatigue, headaches, dizziness, loss of balance, memory problems, joint pain, indigestion, muscle weakness, skin problems, and shortness of breath. This is called Gulf War Syndrome.

There have been a lot of disagreements about whether or not the Gulf War Syndrome is a physical, medical condition. Many believe it to be psychological; the result of serving in combat. Others believe it is the result of exposure to some toxin. Although many ideas exist, the detective work is ongoing.

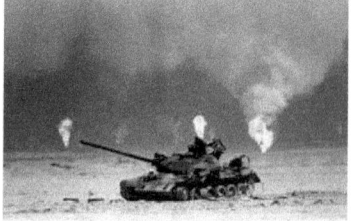

Oil well fires during the first Gulf War

Factors About Environmental Exposures

There are many things found in the environment that may not be good for you. However, our body protects us from most of these toxins. Harm from a toxin depends on several factors:

- Amount of toxin—how much toxin is the person exposed to?
- Toxicity—how dangerous is the toxin?
- Exposure duration—how long a person is exposed?
- Mode of entry—how does the toxin get inside the person?
- Timing—when does the exposure occur (e.g., during pregnancy, childhood, adulthood)?
- Health of the person—the state of the person's health at the time of exposure.
- Genetic makeup—people have differing abilities to deal with an exposure based on their own genetic makeup.

All these factors must be considered at the same time. The impact on people's health varies by type of toxin. Some toxins are deadly in very small amounts, such as botulinum. Foodborne botulism is caused by a bacteria that creates a deadly toxin. This toxin causes paralysis. Because store-bought canned goods are required to be cooked at 121 °C (250 °F) for 3 minutes, it is rare for someone to get botulism from eating store bought food. Home-canned foods with low acid content, such as carrot juice, asparagus, green beans, beets, and corn are more likely to be contaminated with botulin toxin The effects of other toxins depends on the timing of exposure, such as exposure to methylmercury, a form of mercury. The source of methylmercury is eating fish. Mercury seems to accumulate in babies during their time growing inside their mother. Exposure in utero compared to adulthood has much more known serious health effect . For an environmental epidemiologist, figuring out the source of exposure is one step in solving the reason for a disease. Another important step is thinking about other factors that play a role in the occurrence of the disease.

Summary

The relationship between environmental hazards and the health of human communities is of growing concern in the 21st century. The type of pollution source varies from point, area or line source. Whether these sources affect a person's health depends on many factors such as timing of exposure and exposure duration.

Concept Reinforcement

1. In your community, can you give an example of the three sources of pollution?

2. What kind of land was your school built upon? Is there anyway that this land could be contaminated from its past use?

3. What does environmental epidemiology mean to you?

4. Does your community have ozone alert days? How does it affect your life?

Chapter 5 - Psychosocial Epidemiology

Chapter Objectives

- Define psychosocial epidemiology
- Discuss the stress concept as it relates to disease
- Describe examples of the sociocultural influences on health

Psychosocial epidemiology focuses on stress and health. Psychosocial epidemiology also uses surveys to gather data. These surveys ask about knowledge, abilities, attitudes, and personality traits as they are linked to health. Epidemiologists are learning more and more about the importance of non-biological factors and health.

There are many psychosocial factors, such as gender (male or female), age, socioeconomic status (e.g., how rich you are), health risk behaviors (e.g., whether you smoke, drink alcohol or use illegal drugs), life events (e.g., accidents, deaths, moving parental divorce), personality and temperament(inborn personality traits), as well as factors related to the place of work.

Personality, lifestyle and environment can all affect whether a person gets sick or not. A balance between an individual's coping skills and his or her stress level can also be the tipping point of whether one gets sick or not. An individual's belief system can influence the course of a major illness. For example, women with early breast cancer who scored high on helpless measures were more likely to relapse or die within five years of being diagnosed. Psychosocial epidemiologists look for these links.

Examples of Psychosocial Factors and Health

Breast Cancer

Women who have mastectomies with an attitude of "I'm going to beat this" do better than women who have mastectomies and are less positive. Those with a positive attitude live longer and are less likely to have a recurrence of breast cancer. Size of the tumor, the age of the women, or the severity of the illness does not matter.

Cardiovascular Disease (CVD)

Cardiovascular diseases, such as a heart attack, are the leading cause of death and disability in the United States. Type 1 personality—those who are very hard-driving, ambitious, competitive, time-urgent, and unusually quick-tempered and tightly wound, are at an increased risk. Type 1 personality is the first psychosocial factor to be accepted in the medical community as a CVD risk factor.

Cystic Fibrosis (CF)

Cystic Fibrosis is the most common inherited life shortening disease among Caucasians. People with CF live to around 40 years of age. Males live longer than females. One necessary treatment for CF is eating high-fat, high calorie diets. Adolescent girls are less likely to eat this kind of diet. This may be due to societal pressures adolescent feel to stay thin. This may be one partial explanation of the difference in male and female length of survival.

How do Psychosocial Processes Influence Health?

This idea is very complex. The cause and effect path is not straight. For example, smoking cigarettes for decades will significantly increase the chance of getting lung cancer. The path of smoking to lung cancer is straightforward. However, when looking at psychosocial factors, the path is not so straightforward. It may be that some of these psychosocial factors play a role into the length of survival.

Often, psychosocial epidemiology involves diseases that have many risk factors. The influence of each risk factor plays a role. However, we do not yet understand to what degree each factor is important. For example, hypertension, blood lipids, smoking, diet, and personality traits are all known risk factors for heart disease.

Stress

It seems like common sense that stress affects health status. In the late 1960s, scientists described the 10 leading life change events that cause stress. These are:

1. Death of spouse
2. Divorce
3. Marital separation
4. Jail term
5. Death of a close family member
6. Personal injury or illness
7. Marriage
8. Bring fired from a job
9. Marital reconciliation
10. Retirement

The more stressful life events happen, the greater chance a person has of getting sick. Of course, this does not mean that each person will get sick with a life change. It does mean that someone is more likely to get sick. For example, in college, final exam week is very stressful. Some students become sick either during the exam week or immediately after the tests are over. We do not understand why some students get sick and some do not but we do know that stressful events increase the likelihood of getting sick.

Laughter

In contrast to stress, laughter has been shown to be positive. Using humor decreases stress, lessens pain, and improve the quality of a person's life. Some studies have even shown that humor improves a person's ability to fight infection. Dr. Patch Adams believed that laughter, fun and play increased the recovery rate of patients. A movie was made about him.

Summary

Psychosocial epidemiology focuses on the study of stress and health. The key tool used to collect data for psychosocial epidemiology studies is the survey. These surveys collect information about gender, age, socioeconomic status, health risk behaviors, employment, life events, and personality and temperament. Personality, lifestyle, environment, coping skills and stress level all affect whether a person becomes ill. Stress has been shown to contribute to illness, while laughter and positive attitude has been shown to be positive.

Concept Reinforcement

1. What makes figuring out the psychosocial factors associated with disease difficult?

2. What do you think has more impact on one's health, being stressed or being happy? Why?

3. How does one's culture and environment relate to health? Think about the cultural difference between the Western vs non-Western country.

Chapter 6 - Forensic Epidemiology

Chapter Objectives

- Define forensic epidemiology
- Describe who works with epidemiologists
- Provide an example of the use of forensic epidemiology

Forensic epidemiology is a new field. Since the mid-1970s public health and law enforcement officials have worked together on health problems that may have a criminal intent. The term forensic epidemiology was first used in 1999. It describes an expert witness who was an epidemiologist. After the 9/11 event in the fall of 2001, the need for a field called forensic epidemiology was obvious.

The basic definition of forensic is "used in legal proceedings" and the term epidemiology is the study of the distribution and determinants of health related states in specific populations, and the application of this controlled study of health problems. By combining both terms, forensic epidemiology means the use of epidemiologic methods as part of an ongoing investigation or a health problem that may have a criminal intent.

Forensic epidemiology is about epidemiologists and law enforcement working effectively in the event of a threat or attack involving biological or chemical weapons. The primary impact of forensic epidemiology has been in the courtroom. Epidemiologists testify as expert witnesses. More recently, epidemiologists have worked with law enforcement officials in the field, such as during the 2001 anthrax investigation. Anthrax is a serious disease that is caused by bacteria. In the 2001 anthrax investigation, the bacteria was included in envelopes and people who opened the envelope got sick.

In the Courtroom

Epidemiologists are often experts when a case involves environmental exposure and disease or death. Epidemiologists can help explain scientific principles about exposure or explain statistical principles used to figure out the chance of the disease (or death) occurring.

However, science and law are different in basic ways. For example, science is forever changing. The "truths" today may be "falsehoods" tomorrow. Law is final. Epidemiology is the study of populations and not individuals. In court cases, individuals are involved. The court decision is about alleged harm to an individual(s). Law requires a causal link between the exposure and the disease (or death). In epidemiology, it is often impossible to make a 100% link between the exposure and the disease. Even with these differences, epidemiologists are increasingly being used in the courtroom to help with cases.

In the Field

Several legal issues arise when law enforcement officers and epidemiologists work together in the field. Both are interested in protecting the public. However, the rules for each may be different. Areas that may cause problems are:

1. gathering of evidence during public health investigation that is admissible in court
2. access to premises
3. establishing and maintaining a chain of custody of evidence
4. disclosure of confidential health information by public health to law enforcement
5. restricting a person's freedom of movement following exposure to communicable diseases

Let's look at 3 of these legal issues more closely.

Disclosure of Confidential Health Information by Public Health and Law Enforcement

One important part of epidemiology is the protection of human rights. This can be a problem in the case of possible criminal intent to hurt another.

South Dakota Situation with HIV Infection

Epidemiologic research was the leader in determining the link between sexual contact and the spread of HIV. The transmission path is now widely known. Many public health offices provide free HIV testing. However, there are legal issues about this practice. In a widely published case in rural New York State in mid-1997, six young women with newly-diagnosed HIV infection reported having had sexual contact with the same infected man. Using voluntary partner notification and contact tracing, 17 cases of HIV were identified. Publicity surrounding this situation led to legislative attempts to adopt new criminal exposure laws. Although this new law was not adopted in New York, a similar one was adopted in South Dakota.

In South Dakota in 2000, the new law made intentional (knowing) exposure of others to HIV a felony, for which a person could get up to a 15 year prison sentence. One of the first persons found guilty under this law was a college freshman who had sexual intercourse with his girlfriend after he found out he was HIV positive.

However, during the course of this investigation, a major problem arose. The South Dakota health authorities were required to not tell anyone besides the person with HIV about the test results even if they believed that this person was not telling his partners. As a result of this issue, specific language was introduced to allow health officials to disclose this kind of information to law enforcement officers.

> **Tuskegee Syphilis Study**
>
> In 1932, the Public Health Service and the Tuskegee Institute began a project on the natural course of syphilis. They enrolled poor, illiterate black men from rural Alabama (399 with syphilis and 201 without syphilis). Those with syphilis did NOT receive proper treatment when penicillin became the accepted treatment. This is a classic example of violation of human rights in a research setting.

Gathering Admissible Evidence in Public Health Investigators

Even when the situation is very clear, such as the threat in the September 2001 anthrax-laced letter to Senator Tom Daschle. In gathering evidence, law enforcement must comply with the Fourth Amendment prohibition against unreasonable searches and seizures and the Fifth Amendment protection against self-incrimination. Self-incrimination means telling law enforcement information that points the finger at oneself for committing a crime. If a public health official is leading the investigation and does not obtain a search warrant, then it is likely that evidence obtained cannot be used in the court.

Image of the envelope in which the letter containing Anthrax was sent to Senator Tom Daschle during the 2001 anthrax attacks.

The return address given in the top left says: "4th Grade, Greendale School, Franklin Park, New Jersey, 08852." There is no Greendale School at that address, though there is a Greenbrook School in the locality.

Tests conducted at USAMRIID confirmed the presence of fine, "energetic", powdered anthrax within this prestamped 34 cent transmittal envelope. Also present was a one page handwritten letter, clues from which enabled the FBI to create a profile of the sender.

The letter was postmarked at the Hamilton Township postal facility at 5:45 p.m. on October 9 2001. By October 11, it had reached the Brentwood postal facility in Washington which processes US Government mail. Two postal workers, Joseph Curseen Jr. and Thomas Morris Jr., died after contracting inhalational anthrax at the Brentwood facility. The 14,000 square foot facility was decontaminated on December 14, 2002 using chlorine dioxide gas. When it was reopened 26 months after the incident the facility was renamed the "Joseph Curseen Junior and Thomas Morris Junior Processing Distribution Center.

Image courtesy of the FBI

Restricting Freedom of Movement in Response to Public Health Emergencies

In 2003, the SARS outbreak triggered the widest use of quarantine globally since the early 1900s. SARS stands for severe acute respiratory syndrome. In early 2003, SARS spread from China to almost 40 countries around the world. In Canada, almost 20,000 people were kept in home quarantine for 10 days. Only a handful of Canadians refused to stay home. During this time, all their needs, such as food, medicine and work excuses were met by the public officials. In this case, SARS was not purposely given to others. However, forensic epidemiologist and law enforcement worry about other deadly diseases being given to a few people intentionally and then being spread, like SARS spread.

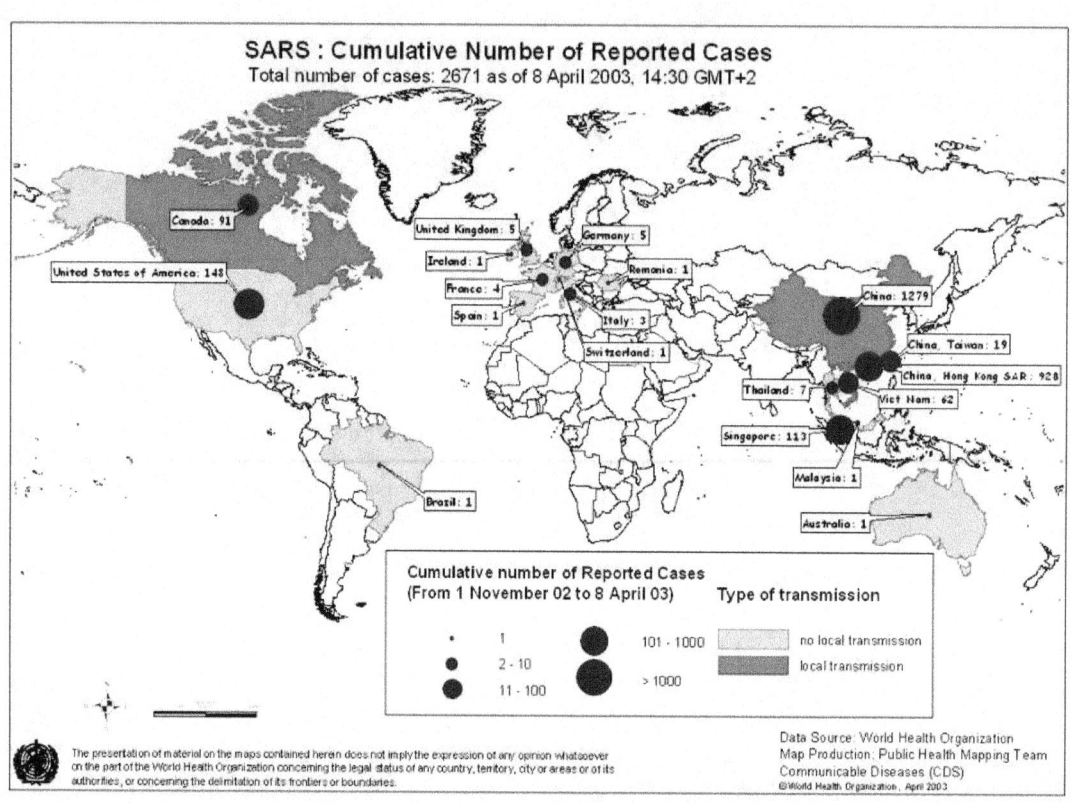

Map of SARS cases from November 1, 2002 to April 8, 2003

Summary

Forensic epidemiology is a new field of study. One characteristic of this field is epidemiologists and law enforcement work together on cases. Both fields involve detective work. In forensic epidemiology, the health outcome has a criminal intent. It did not happen by chance but rather was intentional.

Concept Reinforcement

1. Do you think it is OK to release a name to law enforcement of someone with HIV?

2. Would you support the quarantine of anyone upon flying back home who had traveled to a country with an infectious disease outbreak?

3. Do you think it is reasonable to apply the term "reasonable doubt" to dismiss a case when there will always be less than 100% confidence is an epidemiological finding linking an exposure to a health outcome that was not immediate, such as leukemia?

Chapter 7 - Ecological Study Design

Chapter Objectives

- Define the basic difference between observational and experimental epidemiology
- Describe an ecological study design
- List 2 advantages of an ecological study

Many study designs are available to the epidemiologist. Choosing the appropriate study design depends on many things. In general, the amount of information already known drives the choice of the study design.

Two characteristics of a study will help the epidemiologist pick an observational, quasi-experimental, or an experimental study. Quasi-experimental design means that it looks like an experimental design but one key ingredient is missing—the random assignment of participants. These characteristics are whether the exposure of interest is controlled by the individual and whether the study participants can be randomized.

Exposure of Interest Not Controlled by Individual

Epidemiologists link exposures to health outcomes. For example, epidemiologists showed that smoking is linked with lung cancer. The exposure of interest was smoking. This exposure is controlled by the individual because the individual chooses whether or not to smoke. It would be wrong to have the researcher or government make people smoke in order to study the risks. In a different situation, exposure to air pollution is not controlled by the individual. By living in a city, a person has little control over the air s/he breathes.

Randomization of Participants

Randomization refers to the chance of being assigned to one exposure or not. For example, a participant can be put into a smoking cessation program or not based on the flip of a coin. If the coin lands on heads, the person goes into a new type of smoking cessation program and if the coin lands on tails, the person does not go into this new type of smoking cessation program but rather gets the regular treatment.

Study Type	Exposure of interest controlled by individual	Randomization of participants
Experimental	No	Yes
Quasi-Experimental	No	No
Observational	Yes	No

Study Design

Experimental

A common experimental study design is the randomized controlled trial (RCT). This type of study design is used primarily in research and teaching hospitals. One purpose of an RCT is to test a new drug, therapy or surgical procedure on patients with the disease of interest. Experimental study designs that take place outside of a hospital setting are known as randomized community trials. Community trials are usually about education and behavior change at the population level. Common community trials include smoking cessation programs, physical activity and weight loss programs.

Quasi-Experimental

The second type of study design is quasi-experimental. In this case, the exposure is controlled by the researcher, governmental agency, or even nature. However, unlike RCT, chance does not dictate who is exposed or not. A classic quasi-experimental study involves seat belt use and death from collisions. In this situation, the government controls the exposure—wearing a seat belt or not. If you live in New Hampshire, you do not have to wear a seat belt. However if you live in any other of the 50 states, you are required to wear a seat belt. If we wanted to compare death or injury rate between two states, a person in a state with laws requiring the use of seat belts could not be randomly assigned to wear a seat belt or not. Researchers cannot ask people to break the law. The quasi-experimental design might be comparing deaths from collisions in New Hampshire and Vermont. Even though there may be some people in Vermont who choose to break the law and not wear a seat belt and some people in New Hampshire who choose to wear a seat belt (even though it is not mandated by law), researchers could still look at the statistics comparing the states death rates by motor vehicular injury.

Observational

The third type of study is the observational study. In many situations, an experiment would be wrong. For example, it would be unethical to ask some participants to drink alcohol and drive in town and others to not any drink alcohol and drive in town so that the researcher could study the effects of alcohol consumption on driving ability. Therefore, a lot of epidemiologic research is performed using observational studies. In this situation, patterns of exposure and disease in populations are carefully measured. Two types of observational studies exist: descriptive studies and analytical studies. Descriptive studies look at the person, place, and time to estimate disease frequency and time trends. Analytical studies are used to figure out the reason for a disease. One type of analytical study design is an ecological study.

Ecological Study

The group, not the individual, is the subject of an ecological study. For example, in one study, data on death from breast cancer and the average amount of fat intake per person in 39 countries were collected. Countries with high fat consumption (Netherlands, Denmark, New Zealand, United Kingdom, Canada, United States, etc) also had an increased level of deaths from breast cancer. On the other hand, countries with low fat consumption, such as Thailand, Japan, El Salvador, Ceylon, Philippines, Mexico, Columbia, etc) had many fewer deaths from breast cancer.

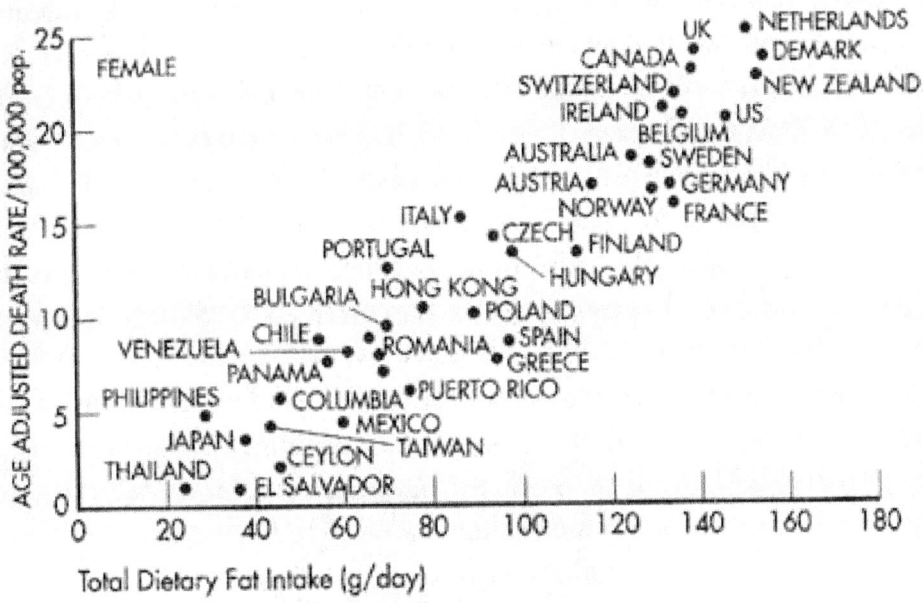

Breast cancer deaths and average fat intake in 39 countries

Once this was shown, the next step was to find out about individual fat consumption and breast cancer risk. In this case, we have not been successful in answering the question. We still do not know if fat consumption is an important risk factor for breast cancer, even after dozens of studies.

Advantages

An ecological study has several benefits:

1. It is generally less expensive than other types of epidemiological studies.

2. It is easy to do since ecological studies often use routinely collected data.

3. It provides ideas about the cause of a disease or condition that can then be further studied using individual level data.

4. It can show researchers new potential risk factors that might not have been thought about before.

Disadvantages

An ecological study has several limitations.

1. Since the ecological study uses routinely collected data, the quality of the data may not be as high as we would like. Poorer quality data can lead to incorrect conclusions

2. Sometimes it is difficult to know if the data really reflect the number of people with the disease, since the criteria for being included in the data may vary.

3. Using the data from an ecological study to say something about individuals. This is known as ecological fallacy. In other words, the misunderstanding occurs when the individual members of the group are thought to have the *average* characteristics of the group.

Ecological Fallacies

One of the main disadvantages is the problem with ecological fallacy. Stereotypes are one form of ecological fallacy. For example if Hawaiians are considered to be good at math, it is an error to think that every Hawaiian is good at math. For any one person in the group of Hawaiians, we do not know their math ability. We only know the average math ability of the group.

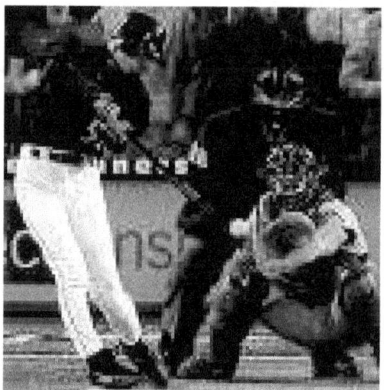

Ichiro Suzuki of the Seattle Mariners

To use a sports example, the batting average of the team will not tell us anything about one player's batting average. For example, the Seattle Mariners' team batting average in October 2008 was 0.265. What was Ichiro Suzuki's batting average? It was much different than 0.265. It was 0.331. If we assumed that Ichiro Suzuki's batting average was the same as the team average, we would have made an ecological fallacy.

Summary

Two key characteristics describe three types of studies. The first key characteristic is whether or not the individual has any control over the exposure. The second characteristic is whether a participant can be randomly assigned to the exposed or unexposed group. Of the analytical study designs, the ecological study designs looks at the group to determine risk factors. One mistake is to apply the findings from an ecological study to an individual. This is known as an ecological fallacy.

Concept Reinforcement

1. Do you think the laws against driving under the influence of alcohol were based on quasi experimental data? If yes, suggest some data.

2. Imagine that your community had an air pollution problem and you are interested in studying asthma. Choose one of the study designs described in this unit and explain how you would study the issue.

3. Are the characteristics that describe your school an ecological fallacy? Explain

Chapter 8 - Cross-sectional Study Design

Chapter Objectives

- Describe a cross-sectional study design

- State the pros and cons of cross-sectional study design

- Explain the concept of correlation

Many study designs are available to the epidemiologist. Choosing the appropriate study design depends on many things. In general, the amount of information already known drives the choice of the study design.

One type of study is observational study. Careful measurement of patterns of exposure and disease in populations are made. Two types of observational studies exist: descriptive studies and analytical studies. Descriptive studies look at the person, place, and time to estimate disease frequency and time trends. Analytical studies are used to figure out the reason for a disease. One type of descriptive study design is cross-sectional study.

Cross-sectional studies observe part of the population at a single point or brief period of time. They often use individual-level data, for example, household interview surveys. A phrase to describe cross-sectional studies is "snap shots". It is a snap-shot since a cross-sectional study captures one picture of the community at one point in time, just like a picture taken with a camera. Typically the cross-sectional studies describe the frequency of health outcomes.

Although cross-sectional studies are limited in their ability to test hypotheses, they can provide insight about the extent of a public health problem. This takes the form of person, place and time.

Cross-sectional studies are useful. One thing that can be figured out from cross-sectional studies is the magnitude of a problem. For example, by gathering data from a survey of college students about drinking more than 5 alcoholic drinks on a single occasion , the severity of the problem can be determined.

Information from cross-sectional studies can be used to focus more research into figuring out why a problem exists. Once a problem is identified, then much more research follows to figure out why. For example, cross-sectionals studies have shown very clearly that the number of children who are obese is increasing every year. A lot of research is being done to figure out why.

Cross-sectional studies can also be used for planning health programs. For example, if a binge problem was discovered in the survey of college students, then universities' health services might start programs to address this problem.

Several national surveys are a cross-sectional study design. In these national surveys, they are repeated. From these data, trends in disease or risk factors can be shown. For example data on adolescents, aged 12-19 years from the National Health Interview Surveys conducted from 1974 – 1991 showed that overall smoking levels went down among that group of adolescents.

Advantages of Cross-sectional Study

A cross-sectional study has several advantages. One advantage is that one study can look at several health issues. In a survey, people can be asked to tell the researcher about their smoking, alcohol drinking, medical conditions, physical exercise, etc. Every one of these topics can be used to show the number of people who smoke, drink alcohol, etc.

Another advantage of cross-sectional study design is the cost. Since the study gathers data over a short period of time, the costs are a lot lower than other study designs.

In cross-sectional studies, participants are contacted once for an exam or interview. This is an advantage since it limits the burden on people; they have to spend less time and energy helping with the research.

Disadvantages of Cross-sectional Study

One disadvantage of a cross-sectional study is that the researcher cannot determine which happened first, the risk factor or exposure versus the disease or illness. Both pieces of information are collected at the same time and it is tough to know which can first.

Cross-sectional studies are not able to look at diseases that are uncommon. When a survey is sent to a community, few respondents are likely to have a rare disease or illness. Therefore, this type of study design is not useful for figuring out trends or frequency of rare diseases or illnesses. Similar, cross-sectional studies are not very help for studying outbreaks or epidemics. By definition the outbreak is a sudden increase in a disease. When cross-sectional survey is mailed to participants, they answer questions about their health and lifestyle choices. Since an outbreak is sudden and unexpected the questionnaire would not ask people whether or not they had that disease.

The third limitation is that cross sectional studies cannot be used to figure out why someone gets a disease, illness or injury. For people in the study that are survivors of a disease, it is difficult to figure out which lifestyle factors are linked to the disease and which are linked to the survival. Cross-sectional studies only describe what exists at the time of contact—at the time of an exam or interview. Hence the name snap-shot.

Finally, cross-sectional studies cannot predict future health events. In repeated cross-sectional surveys, they can show trends but cross-sectional studies cannot be used to figure out why these trends happen. Therefore cross-sectional studies cannot predict.

Analysis of Cross-sectional Survey Data

One way to describe the relation between a risk factor and disease outcome is to use a statistical technique called correlation. This term means there is an association between two variables where the fluctuation in the values of each of the variables shows a pattern that is unlikely to occur by chance.

A few graphs might make this clear.

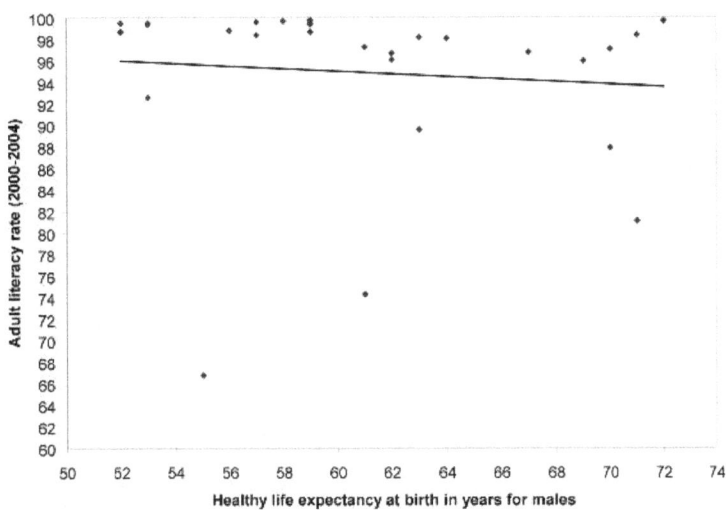

Weak negative correlation: Adult literacy rates and healthy life expectancy at birth in years for males

This graph shows that men in some countries who are slightly less educated are likely to have a slightly longer healthy life. When approximately 96% of the male population is literate, they live fewer years than when approximately 92% of the male population is literate.

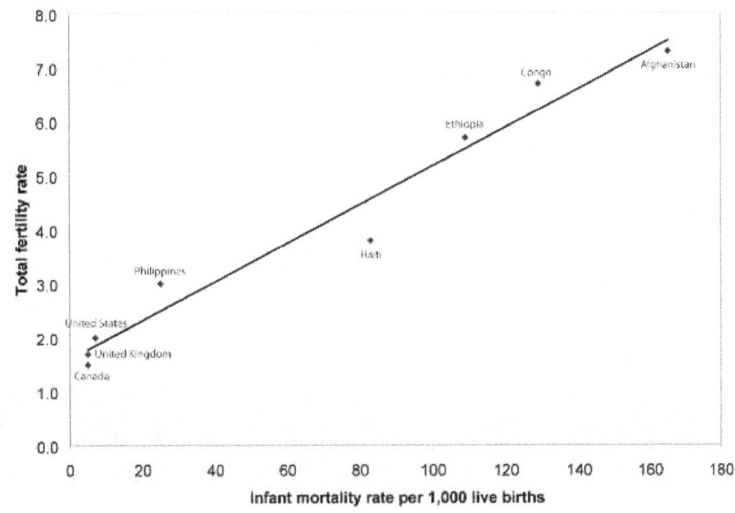

Strong positive correlation: Infant mortality rate and fertility rate in eight countries

This shows that a higher infant death rate is linked with having more children.

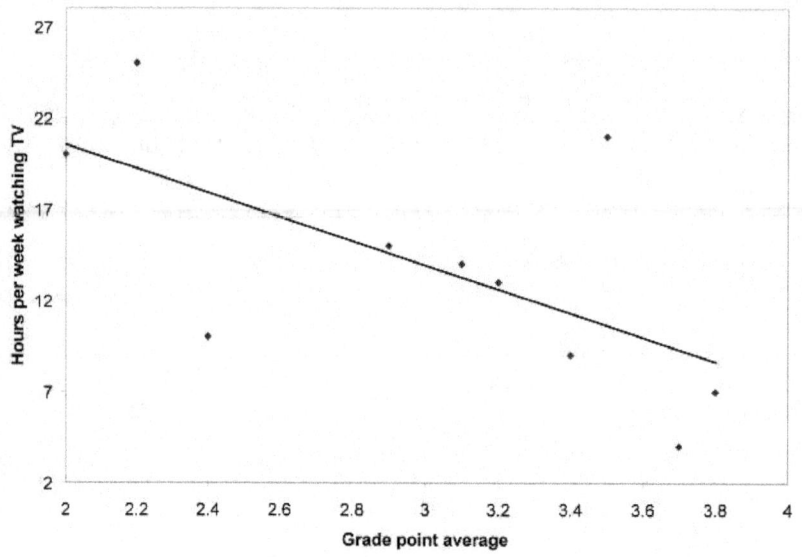

Strong negative correlation: Number of hours watching TV and grade point average

This shows that watching TV less is linked to better grades.

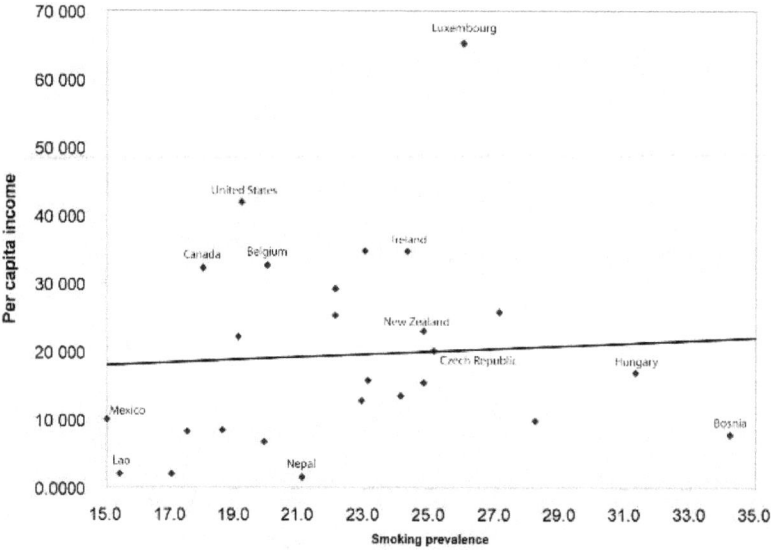

Weak positive correlation: percent smoking and per capita income in selected countries from 2004 WHO data

This shows that a higher proportion of smokers, age 15 and older, are slightly more likely to have a higher income in selected countries.

Just as a reminder, a correlation does not mean that one of the two "causes" a change in the other. In addition, these data are about the population. They do not tell us anything about an individual.

Summary

Of the study designs available to the epidemiologist, one of the most common is cross-sectional design. Cross-sectional study design is an observational study. It characterizes the population at a single point in time. Correlations are often used to show the relation between two factors in a cross-sectional study.

Concept Reinforcement

1. What would be interesting factors to gather about your school to be able to create a snapshot about athletic injury.

2. What kind of correlation do you think exists between high school students playing sports and weight?

3. What kind of correlation do you think exists between amounts of time a babies cries and the amount of time a baby is held?

Chapter 9 - Case-control Study Design

Chapter Objectives

- Describe a case-control study design
- Define a case and a control participant
- Define recall bias

One of the underlying principles of all study designs is that disease does not occur randomly, but rather there is an underlying causal pathway to the disease. Of the many types of study designs, the case-control study design first identifies two groups—those with the disease and those without the disease. The case-control study seeks to identify possible causes of the disease by determining how these two groups differ with regard to exposures.

Case-control studies are considered retrospective. Retrospective means that in the study, the disease or health outcome is identified first and then the epidemiologist works backward to try and figure out what is associated with the disease or health outcome. This backward looking work is accomplished by asking participants about lifestyle habits and exposures at specific time points in the past. For example, "When you were a child, did your parents or others who lived with you smoke in the house?" Another retrospective question might be "How old were you when you started smoking cigarettes regularly?"

Recall Bias

One concern about case-control studies is recall bias. Recall bias means that people in the different groups remember things differently. Intuitively, this makes sense. When people are diagnosed with a disease, it is natural for them to try to figure out why. They will often think very hard about their past. They will try to find some reason why they got the disease and not someone else. In addition, they may also research about their disease and note the risk factors. Consequently, their recall of past events may be different from someone who has never had the disease.

For example, let's say that a disease is due to being around clothes during adolescence that were dry cleaned. Dry cleaned clothes emit cleaning fluid odors for a few days. The case-control study is figuring out if exposure to fumes from dry cleaning chemical are linked to the disease. Study participants are asked in a survey about being around dry cleaning in the home during adolescents ("when you were a teenager…"). Because there were some articles about the possibility of this chemical's link to the disease, some of the cases had thought about this possibility. These cases asked their parents and investigated their exposure before they ever received a questionnaire. In contrast, for the controls, the first time they were asked to think about this possibility was when they read the question in the survey. They answered the question on the spot without investigating the possibility. For example, they did not call up their parents and ask about this. In this example, even though the same number of cases and controls were really exposed to fumes that come off the dry

---

Diethylstilboestrol (DES) Illustration

A classic case-control study was launched with only 8 young women who had been diagnosed with an extremely rare vaginal cancer in one hospital. In 1971, Herbst and Scully reported that 8 cases of an extremely rare vaginal cancer and 32 matched controls were interviewed about possible risk factors. They found that all cases' mothers had taken the synthetic estrogen called diethylstilboestrol (DES). DES had been prescribed to pregnant women since 1947 under the mistaken belief that DES would prevent spontaneous abortions (miscarriages). Seven months after this publication, the US Food and Drug Administration withdrew approval for use of DES by pregnant women. Research continues on daughters and sons of mothers who took DES. These adult children have several health problems that are linked to DES exposure.

cleaned clothes, the cases were more likely to remember the situation. They more often reported an exposure than a control. This led to the researchers reporting a link between the chemical emitted from dry cleaned clothes and the disease. But this link was not really there. It was due to the recall bias.

To review, in case-control studies, cases have the disease. Controls do not have the disease. Information about the people with the disease (cases) is compared to people without the disease (controls). Case-control study design is the appropriate choice for rare diseases. Remember, the disease is first selected and data for many characteristics and exposures of the participants are then collected. Consequently, many possible risk factors for the disease can be studied since this information is collected in the survey.

Enrollment Process – Selection of Cases and Controls

For the selection of cases, the researcher first defines a case. Once this has been determined, the researcher needs to figure out how to enroll these cases.

Misclassification

The reason these factors are important is the issue of misclassification. Misclassification means that someone is thought to be a case (has the disease) but is really not a case. On the other hand, misclassification can also mean someone is a control (does not have the disease) and is not really a control. For example, we want to study the risk factors associated with drinking alcohol in pregnant women. Since most women do not realize they are pregnant until about 4 – 6 weeks after conception, some women may say they are not pregnant at enrollment when they really are pregnant. This is an example of misclassification. Some controls are really cases. They were classified incorrectly.

Another way that misclassification can occur is if the definition of a case is too broad, there may be some people assigned to the case population who do not have the disease. On the other hand, if the definition of a case is too restrictive, there may not be enough cases to conduct the study. Because of the importance of minimizing misclassification, when given a choice, the researcher would prefer the case definition be more restrictive than less.

Finding Cases and Controls

Case ascertainment (identification of cases) rests on the concept that all cases have an equal chance of entering the study. However, there are few lists that contain all cases, such as a cancer registry. Another source of cases is patients who go to a hospital for treatment. One of the concerns about using hospitals is that it is likely the most severe cases are seen at these places and the distribution of risk factors may be atypical. Consequently, results from this type of study may not provide results that can be applied to any situation.

Selection of controls is also very important. One fundamental characteristic of the control population is that the controls have the same characteristics of the cases (except for the exposure of interest). In other words, the controls are the same as the cases in all respects other than the disease and the risk factors of interest. The underlying concept in a case-control study is that the cases are presumed to have the disease because of an excess or deficiency of an exposure, compared to the controls. Usually, proportions of cases and controls in 5-year age groups, males and female, different races, educational levels are characteristics that researchers want to be similar for both populations and only the risk factor of interest different.

Determining the number of controls in a case-control is part of a power calculation, which is beyond the scope of this chapter. Suffice to say, many case-control studies use equal numbers of cases and controls. However, the maximum statistical power would be to use four controls for every case. Determination of the number of controls for a study is often influenced by cost and available funding. Sometimes case ascertainment is very expensive whereas control identification is much less expensive. Therefore, a researcher may chose to enroll more controls than cases.

Identifying controls that come from the same population at risk for the disease or condition is a guiding principal. Several sources of controls are available with each source have inherent strengths and weaknesses. The researcher needs to carefully weigh the strengths and limitations of each source.

Advantages and Disadvantages of Case-control Study

As with all study designs, there are several strengths and limitation of the case-control study design.

Advantages of Case-control Study

One reason to use the case-control study design is that a researcher can focus on a rare disease. The cases are those with a rare disease. The controls are those without the rare disease. Cancer is considered a rare disease. Studies about infectious disease choose case-control study design.

Another advantage of case-control study design is that it takes a short period of time to collect the data. This is helpful in moving forward in understanding the risk factors associated with a disease. This type of study is also relatively easy to collect data. A survey is sent to participants or participants are called and asked about risk factors. In some situations, the participant is asked to give the researcher a biospecimen such as a sample of blood, urine, fingernail or toenail, or saliva. These biospecimens are measures for a specific reason that is linked to a risk factor.

The size of the study is relatively small. The number of participants is usually hundreds to thousands versus thousands to tens of thousands. The number of participants is closely linked to the cost of the study. Consequently, the relatively low cost of this study design is also a strength.

Disadvantages of Case-control Study

One of the major limitations of a case-control study is the retrospective design. Remember this means that participants are asked about exposures and lifestyle habits that happened to them in the past.

Another disadvantage of a case-control study is the uncertainty of the timing of the exposure and the disease. At what time in the life of the individual was the exposure important—-during growth in the womb, during adolescence, during young adulthood, during menopausal changes for women, during later life, etc. The timing of the exposure is almost never known and participants are almost never asked about exposure at all the important periods of life.

A final limitation of the study design is having controls that really like the cases except for the disease of interest. On paper it seems really easy to selecting the cases and controls for the study, but in reality, this is much more difficult. Real differences beyond the risk factors of interest between these groups can limit the usefulness of the findings.

Summary

One common type of observational study design is the case-control study. The cases are identified and their risk factors are compared to the controls. Cases are people with the disease or illness and controls are people without the disease or illness. For the case-control study design, first the disease or illness is known. Second the researcher asks participants about their lifestyle choices, exposures and behaviors before the disease. Because participants have to remember information that happened in the past, there is a possibility that the recall will be different between cases and controls. This is known as recall bias.

Concept Reinforcement

1. What is an example of recall bias?

2. Where would you go in your community to enroll cancer cases?

3. If you asked your aunt or uncle or grandparent about their exposure to DDT, an insecticide commonly used in the 1970s, do you think they would remember it? Why don't you try.

Chapter 10 - Cohort Study Design

Chapter Objectives

- Describe a cohort study design
- List 2 questions that could be asked using a cohort study design
- Describe the differences between a prospective and retrospective study

A cohort is a group of people that have a common characteristic that is followed over a period of time. An occupational cohort is made up of people who share an exposure in a specific setting. The other type of cohort is one in which the participants share a non-specific exposure and have a general commonality, such as a cohort made up of nurses. A cohort study design is an observational study design. In a cohort study design, data is collected from the cohort at least two times.

Types of Cohort Studies

Cohorts can be studied either forward in time (prospectively) or backward in time (retrospectively). In the prospective cohort study, the variable of interest is measured *before* the health outcome has occurred. In contrast, for a retrospective cohort study, the historical cohort is reconstructed with exposure status determined from past records and data on the outcome of interest is determined at the start of the study. In both the prospective and retrospective cohort study design, the researcher is comparing exposed and unexposed groups. The key difference between the two study designs is the calendar time. In the prospective cohort study design, the exposure and non-exposure are determined as they occur during the study years. Before the exposure status is figured out, the health outcome of interest is identified in the cohort. In the retrospective cohort study design, the exposure is determined from historic records and the disease status is typically figured out at the start of the study.

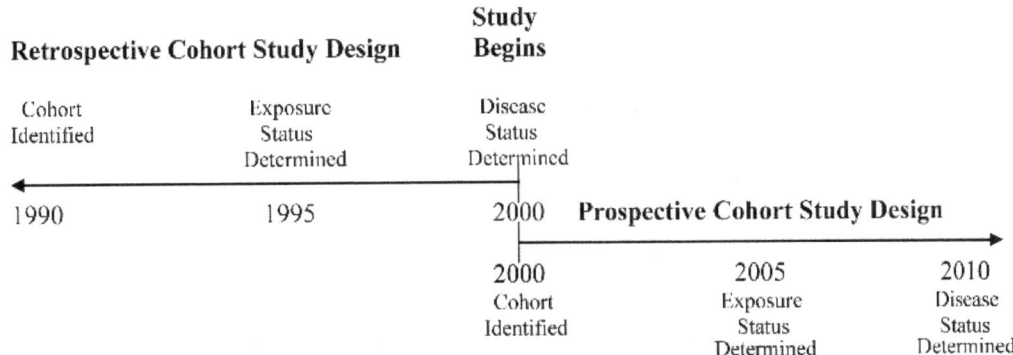

Timeline for retrospective and prospective cohort study designs

> **Prospective cohort study: Framingham Heart Study.**
>
> Cardiovascular disease (CVD) is the leading cause of death and serious illness in the United States, yet little was known about the risk factors associated with CVD when the Framingham Heart Study was launched in 1948. The objective of the study was to identify common factors or characteristics associated with CVD by following 5,209 men and women ages 30-61 who had not developed overt symptoms of CVD, suffered a heart attack or stroke from the town of Framingham, Massachusetts. In 1971, a second-generation (offspring) cohort of 5,124 of the original participants' adult children and their spouses were enrolled. Currently, a third generation of participants (children of the Offspring Cohort) is being enrolled. The Generation III Cohort's goal is to enroll 3,500 grandchildren of the original cohort. Over the years the Framingham Heart Study has led to the identification of major CVD risk factors including high blood pressure, high blood cholesterol, smoking, obesity, diabetes, and physical inactivity.

Enrollment Process

The researcher identifies a population (cohort) of interest. For example, in the Nurses' Health Study, the researchers selected female registered nurses as the cohort. In 1976, 121,700 nurses ages 30-55 completed the first survey.

At the time of enrollment, the researcher figured out the exposure status and other characteristics of the cohort. For the Nurses' Health Study, researchers were interested in the relation of hormonal factors, a variety of nutrients, diabetes, exercise, and brand of cigarettes smoked with subsequent risk of coronary heart disease, pulmonary embolism, and stroke. A pulmonary embolism is a clot in the lungs.

The researchers follow the cohort over time with data collection every couple of years. They were able to identify women who had the health outcome of interest in the exposed and unexposed group. In the Nurses' Health Study cohort, exposure information was collected every two years. Very few women dropped out of the study. As of 2008, the nurses are still being followed. One hallmark of a cohort study is a lengthy follow up period.

Selecting the Cohort

A basic requirement in selecting the cohort for a particular health outcome rests on the concept that everyone in the cohort is at risk for that particular health outcome.

Another is no one in the cohort at the start of the study has that particular health outcome. Consequently, figuring out who is part of the cohort depends on the particular health outcome the researcher is interested in studying.

Obviously, the concept of population at risk for the health outcome implies that only people who are alive at the time of cohort enrollment are eligible to be part of the cohort. This is the third requirement.

These three criteria for selecting a cohort: (1) at risk for the health outcome, (2) free of the health outcome of interest, and (3) alive. However, other important criteria for selecting a cohort might not make it so straightforward. For example, if a researcher wants to study polio, who should be in the cohort? Would an individual who received the vaccine be included or excluded? If the polio vaccine gave 100% prevention, then by definition this individual would not be at risk of getting polio. However, it is unlikely that anyone could reasonably argue that having a polio vaccine gives complete and total protection from this disease. So the eligibility criteria may not be as simple as first thought.

Population-based Study Participants

In a population-based cohort study, the cohort involves either the entire population or a representative sample of the population. One example of a population-based cohort is the Framingham Heart Study. People aged 30-61 and residents of Framingham, Massachusetts joined the study. Of the town's population of 28,000, the study had enrolled 6,500 randomly selected residents. In this type of study, the participants were not selected based on an exposure or risk factor for a disease, nor did they have differing levels of exposure.

Exposure-based Study Participants

Rare exposures cannot be studied using cohort study. For example, it would take a cohort of at least 1,000,000 children to study childhood cancer using cohort study design because childhood cancer is a rare disease.

Using a population that we think has enough exposure that is linked to a disease or illness is another way to select participants. An occupational cohort is a common source of study participants. Exposure on the job often means that workers are exposed to much higher levels than the general public. For example, people working in a lead mine, are likely to have much higher levels of lead exposure than the general public.

Advantages and Disadvantages of a Prospective Cohort Study

Several advantages are associated with a cohort study. One of the most prominent is the establishment of a sequential order of events. In other words, first the exposure is identified and then, after some passage of time, the health outcome is determined. This type of study design eliminates recall bias since exposure data is obtained in real time and is not something that the study participants have to recall. Another advantage of a cohort study is that several health outcomes can be explored at the same time and over the course of the study. In the Framingham Heart study, blood pressure and cholesterol levels were two of several risk factors of cardiovascular disease that were evaluated.

Because of the lengthy follow up required, usually years or decades, several difficulties can arise. One difficulty is continued funding of the study. The National Institutes of Health typically award grants for a maximum of 5 years. Consequently, for the Framingham Study that has been actively collecting data for over 60 years, a dozen grant applications have had to be awarded. With each grant application, a chance of rejection exists since the amount of money available to all researchers is limited. Further, it is possible that the cohort will outlive the principal investigator (PI). For example in the National Children's Study, a cohort of 100,000 children will be followed to age 21. The enrollment of the cohort will take over 10 years. Consequently, if a PI is age 50 at the launch of the study which will be launched in 2009, it is unlikely that the PI will still be in active research and may not even be alive 30 years later, when the data from the completed study are ready for analyses. Of course, for this study, there will be numerous results along the way for the current researchers.

Another concern with cohort studies is the difficulty of retaining study participants. Several scenarios exist in which the number of participant who begins the study is less than the number of participants who finish the study. This is known as loss to follow up. One scenario is that study participants can not be located at the next contact period. Participants can opt out of continuing with the study and participants can die during the study period. As a general rule of thumb, the validity of the study requires that losses to follow up, for whatever reason, not exceed 20%. During the enrollment period, not enrolling those who are deemed likely to not remain in the study, providing incentives for each contact, having periodic contact not related to data collection activities are all strategies to minimize loss to follow up.

A cohort usually requires a very large sample size (Framingham Heart Study, which is considered a relatively small cohort study, initially enrolled 6,500 participants and the National Children's Study plans to enroll 100,000 children). The large study size translates into significant study expenses. In addition, detecting rare diseases is not a common goal of cohort studies.

Summary

Cohort study design is comprised of participants who share a common characteristic. This observational study design collects data from participants at lease two times over a period of time. Many cohorts lasts years and a few have been going on for decades. One of the main advantages of a cohort study is the sequence of exposure and then disease is clear. Cost of the study and maintaining contact with all participants over the course of the study are two limitations of cohort studies.

Concept Reinforcement

1. What is the key difference between a retrospective and prospective cohort study design?

2. What could be the characteristics of a community that would lead to loss to follow up due to "unable to locate?"

3. What would be an appropriate cohort to study use of electronic communication on career choices?

Chapter 11 - Randomized Controlled Trial (RCT) Study Design

Chapter Objectives

- Describe a randomized controlled trial study design

- Describe the reason for using a placebo

- Describe the reason for blinding in a RCT

Of the epidemiological study designs, experimental designs allow researchers to understand the cause of diseases. In the experimental design, the researcher attempts to change only one thing between the two groups. One type of experimental study design is called randomized controlled trial.

A randomized controlled trial is called a randomized clinical trial when the setting is a medical facility. This type of RCT typically investigates a pharmaceutical medication intervention (a new drug), some type of treatment intervention (a new treatment), or some type of screen (a test used to detect a disease in individuals without signs or symptoms of the disease) for a disease in a clinical setting. The unit of analysis is the individual. For randomized community trial, one group of people or one community receives an intervention and the other group or community does not. The unit of analysis is the group or community.

The Enrollment Process

There are three steps to launching a RCT. First, the reference population is determined. In other words, who is supposed to benefit from the intervention? This is the population to which the researcher hopes to generalize his/her findings.. The next step involves defining the experimental population. This is a practical representation of the population. For randomized clinical trials, patients seen by the appropriate doctors associated with hospitals involved in clinical trials are often the experimental population. For randomized community trials, residents of the community are the experimental group. Volunteers are enrolled from the experimental population who meet the eligibility criteria. The last step in launching a RCT is random allocation of the volunteers to the treatment group or the control group. The treatment group will receive the intervention whereas the control group will not receive this intervention. One ethical aspect of receiving treatment is that the control group will receive the gold standard of currently accepted standard patient care, if appropriate.

Randomization

Randomization means that chance alone determines whether a participant is assigned to the treatment group or the control group. Why is randomization such an important characteristic of RCT? A couple of benefits are gained from randomization. One benefit is that subjective bias of the investigators, either overt or covert, is not introduced into study design. This means that the researchers do not influence the results of the study, either knowingly or by some action that they are not necessarily aware they are doing. For example, a study was carried out in New York City to test a tuberculosis vaccine in the mid 20th century. Physicians were instructed to divide their eligible pediatric patients into two groups, intervention and control groups. The intervention group received the TB vaccine. At the end of the study, it was discovered that the physicians selected children for treatment based on the parent's intelligence and cooperative nature. Controls were comprised of children of less intelligent and non-cooperative parents. This non-random allocation of eligible patients may have influenced the study results since one could argue that cooperative parents may be more health conscious, seek medical advice, and therefore have their children at a lower risk for TB in general. Another benefit of randomization is that the investigator hopes that the two groups are comparable with regard to characteristics such as average age, sex, race, severity of the disease, etc. However, randomization is a chance event. Consequently, randomization does not guarantee comparability because the groups will not be matched by specific characteristics, though with larger sample size the likelihood of comparability increases. This likelihood is a statistical truth. In randomization from one population, the larger the sample size, the more likely the groups will look alike. For example, imagine randomly selecting 10 students from a large high school of 1500 students. The average age of these 10 students are less likely to match the average age of the student body than if 500 students were randomly selected.

Ethical Considerations

Because a RCT enrolls people and, depending on the intervention, a RCT enrolls sick people, several ethical considerations need to be addressed.

1. The treatment options should be at least as good as other treatment options based on previous randomized controlled trials. If a good standard of treatment exists, this should be given to the controls. One rule in medicine is that the patient's welfare is the most important consideration. Consequently, it would be unethical to subject patients to an inferior treatment or no treatment, if one exists.

2. The hypothesis under study in a RCT should be of clinical significance and be useful for future patients.

3. Informed consent is vital for a RCT to be ethical. There are numerous examples of unethical studies because the patients were not informed. A component of informed consent is the ability to opt out of the study. The medical experiments performed on prisoners of war during WW II are examples of unethical research.

4. The entire group of participants should be recruited in a timely manner. Having patients assigned to the intervention group means they are not receiving the current gold standard of treatment during the course of the study. It is unethical to put these patients on the waiting list until a sufficient number of patients are enrolled if the waiting time is unreasonable.

Blinding

Once the study population has been identified and assigned to the intervention or control group, measurements are taken of both groups to determine the influence of the treatment. The monitoring of patients for 1) occurrence of events that the intervention is suppose to prevent, 2) occurrence of unexpected results or 3) end of the illness. Specific protocols are used and followed meticulously so that bias is not introduced in the study.

In a single-blind study, the participants do not know whether they are given the treatment or not. In a double-blind study, not only are the participants kept in the dark about the kind of treatment they are receiving, but the study staff do not even know who is in the treatment and control groups. Blinding is used to minimize the placebo effect. A placebo effect is any benefit from treatment with an inert substance (inert means not chemically active), such as a sugar pill instead of a medication. For the study staff, this placebo effect might be seen in how the study staff treats the patients based on group status. In some situations, it is unethical to have patients participate in blinded studies, such as a surgical intervention because it is unethical to have the control undergo a fake surgery.

Noncompliance

Once the RCT has been designed, participants enrolled, and intervention blinded, if possible, the next issue that may greatly influence the study results is noncompliance. Noncompliance can take two forms: dropouts and drop-ins. Those who do not fully comply with the treatment protocol are known as noncompliant. In some cases, patients decided to stop participating in the trial during the course. This is also known as noncompliance. The other form of noncompliance happens when the control group inadvertently takes the agent under study. This happened in a heart attack study in which aspirin was used for the treatment group. Many over-the-counter preparations contain aspirin and some of the controls took these over-the-counter preparations. Most RCTs have noncompliance issues. However, statistical tests are used to deal with this issue so that even with poor compliance, the results of the RCT can be published.

Advantages and Disadvantages of a RCT

The biggest advantage of a RCT is that the study results provide strong evidence since detailed information can be collected at the start of the study and throughout the study. Part of that advantage is the ability of RCTs to control for other factors that might influence the study results by carefully selecting participants. Another advantage is that dose levels can be predetermined by the researcher.

The major disadvantage of a RCT is the cost of the study. For pharmaceutical medicine, it can cost millions of dollars to bring a new drug to the market. These pharmaceutical drugs have to go through 4 phases of clinical trials.

1. Phase 1 clinical trial begins testing the new drug on a small number of people. Usually the people are healthy. The purpose of phase 1 trial is to look at the safety of the drug in people and start to figure out the proper dose.

2. Phase 2 clinical trial takes the drug testing to the next phase. Up to 200 people are used for Phase 2 trials. The safe and effective dose is figured out. Side effects are also determined.

3. Phase 3 clinical trials are the first trial with randomization. Hundreds to thousands of people are randomized to those in the intervention group or the control group. The intervention group is compared to the normal treatment.

4. Phase 4 clinical trials move the drug into the general population. Physicians can prescribe the drug to patients. Safety surveillance continues during phase 4.

RCTs are generally labor intensive, which translates into a high cost per patient. Consequently, most the sample size of most RCTs is constrained. This means that large effects can be observed, but not modest or small effects. Another disadvantage of a RCT is the issue of compliance. If there is a problem with compliance, the study findings may be weakened. Often RCTs take a long period of time to reach a conclusion.

Randomized controlled trials are considered the gold standard in epidemiology since they are robust experimental designs. The strength of the findings from a RCT far surpasses those of other designs. Several components of a RCT must be adhered to for it to be useful. Whether the findings in a RCT can be applied to the general population and ethical concerns are major considerations in RCT.

Summary

The experimental design of RCT allows researchers to control over who receives the exposure as well as the level of exposure. The researchers can more confidently state a cause-effect relationship with a RCT than observational study designs. Although RCTs are costly and take considerable time to complete, the findings provide strong evidence. No medication can be put on the market without going through randomized clinical trials.

Concept Reinforcement

1. Although both randomized clinical trials and randomized community trials are both experimental in design, what are differences between the two?

2. Why is randomization important?

3. If the study was not blinded, do you think the compliance issues would be different? Explain.

Chapter 12 - Surveillance and Mortality Data

Chapter Objectives

- Define surveillance
- Explain the use of ICD
- State the pros and cons of death certificates variables
- State the pros and cons of the underlying cause of death from death certificates

Surveillance is the continuous collection of descriptive information about the population. It is done is a step-by-step way. These data are analyzed, interpreted, and disseminated. The fundamental purpose of surveillance is to monitor health. Often surveillance data are used to shape public policy.

A Brief History

One of the very first collection of health statistics was in England, by John Graunt in a publication called *Natural and Political Observations Made Upon the Bills of Mortality*. This publication summarized causes of death in London in 1662. One of his contributions was discovering regularities in medical and social phenomena.

Since early settlers in the New World were mostly English, they were used to registering christenings, marriages and burials. Beginning in the mid 1600s, all English parishes were required to collect these data. When the settlers came to America, they continued the practice of recording births, deaths and marriages at the local churches. However, these data were not complete or often used. The fear of cholera played an important role in encouraging state legislative action to put in place a system for accurate registration of births and deaths (registries) in some major American cities in the middle of the 19th century. The U.S. Census, under the directive of President Theodore Roosevelt, began an annual collection of vital statistics from these registries and by the later half of the 20th century, birth and death registries throughout the United States were providing accurate data. However, marriage and divorce data have yet to be sent to the State registrar in all 50 states (approximately ¾ of the states send marriage license data to State registrars and approximately ½ of the states send in divorce decrees to the State registrars.)

Birth Certificates

The birth certificate data collection process was automated to a standard set of data in 2002. Most states have both electronic and paper birth certificates. The plan is for all states have electronic birth certificates by 2012.

In reality, an employee of the hospital where a baby is born typically fills out the birth certificate. Since these people are usually not researchers, they do not always understand the importance of gathering accurate data. It is well known that the smoking and alcohol answers are not reliable data because mothers may be embarrassed to admit the truth. Sometimes the employee will ask the mother, "You didn't smoke during pregnancy, did you?" Can you see how the phrasing of this question introduces bias and would encourage the mother to agree with the data collector even if the truth was different? Race is another data point that is not very reliable on the birth certificate since the data collector may fill in whatever s/he thinks is the baby's race and ethnicity based on their own observation.

Death Certificates

One of the first accounts of a systematic analysis of health was John Graunt's work on the causes of deaths in London in 1662. In hindsight it is easy to understand why mortality data would be an excellent tool for understanding population health in the 17th century. It was surveillance data in which no one could be misclassified; death is an obvious state. Some of the data in the records would have given accurate details, such as seasonal variations in deaths, infant mortality rates, and excess of male deaths compared to females. Other data would have been less accurate, particularly results using the underlying cause of death (UCOD) variable since specific diagnoses of diseases and illness were far from accurate.

Underlying Cause of Death

Underlying cause of death means the cause of death is the disease or complications that caused the death. All death certificates have data fields called "cause of death" and "underlying causes of death" (UCOD). It is not the mode of dying, such as a cardiac arrest. The underlying causes of death are defined as the disease or injury which started the train of events leading directly or indirectly to death or the circumstances of the accident or violence which produced the fatal injury.

These days the law requires reporting of deaths to the National Center for Health Statistics. Doctors, coroners, medical examiners and funeral home directors fill out death certificates. The National Center for Health Statistics is working on improving the quality of the data, particularly the underlying cause of death. As you can imagine, the true cause of death may not always be recorded, such as in the case of a suicide. In other situations, figuring out the underlying cause of death may not be straightforward, particularly when an individual has several medical conditions.

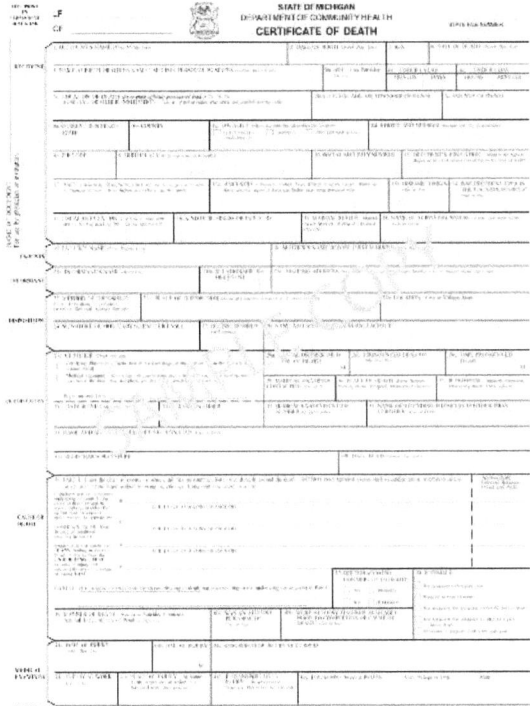

Death certificate form from Michigan

Classification of Death

First introduced in 1893 by Jacques Bertillon, a classification system for cause of death has been revised every ten years by the World Health Organization (WHO) and the coding has been published in the "*Manual of International Statistical Classification of Diseases, Injuries and Causes of Death (ICD)*. It is in its 10th version. The ICD has become the most widely used classification system in the world.

The ICD has been revised approximately every 10 years since 1900. These revisions reflect advances in the medical field, changes in our understanding of disease mechanisms and terminology, and are designed to maximize the amount of information and flexibility a code can provide.

Changes in disease definition will not only impact the ICD coding but also the UCOD on the death certificate. For example on January 1, 1993, the acquired immunodeficiency syndrome (AIDS) definition was expanded from the original definition published in 1987 to one that included all human immunodeficiency virus (HIV)-infected persons with certain diseases. With this change in definition, there was a 204% increase in number of reported cases in the first 3-months of 1993 compared to the same time period in the previous year. A larger fraction of people with AIDS who die will have this diagnosis subsequently listed as the UCOD.

Data Quality

In any type of surveillance system, the quality of the data is important. Accuracy is important. Is the underlying cause of death correct? How about the race of the baby on the birth certificate? Besides accuracy, two other key aspects of data quality are completeness and timeliness. Completeness means that all the cases *and* their respective information are represented in the dataset. Timeliness means the cases diagnosed are represented in the dataset soon after diagnosis (e.g., within a couple of months). If the data quality is untrustworthy, then some analyses cannot be done. For example, it is well known that the population estimate of number of Hispanic births is under-reported due to the misclassification mentioned above. Therefore, analyzing data by race may not give accurate results.

Functionality of Mortality Data Analysis

Mortality data can serve many functions.

1. One function of a mortality study is to evaluate the effectiveness of a new screening technique. For example, mammography are a screening test for breast cancer The key point of information the researcher searches for is the following: "Did more, the same, or less people die of the disease in which the screening test was used compared to those who did not have the screening test?"

2. Mortality data can also be a useful indicator of severity of the disease from both the clinical and public health perspective.

3. Mortality data can also be used to indicate disease risk, if the number of people who die from the disease is high and survival time from diagnosis to death is short. Pancreatic cancer is an example in which the mortality data also reflects the disease risk. The prognosis for someone diagnosed with pancreatic cancer is about 3 months.

Summary

One function of epidemiology for hundreds of years has been the collection of health data. From these data, the health of the population can be described. Birth and death certificates are collected today. The quality of the elements in the birth and death certificate is improving. With high quality records, much can be learned about the health of a community.

Concept Reinforcement

1. If one of the three characteristics of quality data was poor, what would be the consequence?

2. Currently, only births and deaths are collected by all states. What do you think the advantage would be of collecting records of divorces.

3. If you had the money, what surveillance data would you collect in every state?

Chapter 13 - Screening

Chapter Objectives

- Explain the difference between diagnostic and screening tests

- Define the characteristics of a good screening test

- List the criteria to consider before the implementation of a national screening program

A fundamental belief in public health is the best approach to health care is prevention. This is known as primary prevention. However if all cases of a disease cannot be prevented, the next best approach is called secondary prevention. Secondary prevention is to identify those who do not have any symptoms of the disease or are in an early stage of the disease through screening. The purpose of screening is to reduce morbidity and death by catching the disease early. Early detection of diseases is often linked with longer life. The final stage of prevention is called tertiary prevention. Tertiary prevention is limiting the progression of the disease. An example of tertiary prevention is giving antiretroviral therapy for people diagnosed with HIV. The antiretroviral therapy does not cure anyone; but it does slow the progression of HIV to full blown AIDs.

In this chapter we are going to explore the characteristics of secondary prevention in the form of screening practices.

As stated above, the purpose of screening is to catch the disease or illness in an early stage. There are many kinds of screening tests used to determine health status. For instance, all newborns have a mandatory newborn screening test that evaluates 29-50 conditions. Blood pressure is another example of a screening test that all adults get during their physical examination.

There is often confusion between screening and diagnosis. Screening usually occurs in people who do not have any symptoms and are not suspected of having the disease. Diagnostic tests are used to confirm whether someone has a disease or not. Sometimes the screening test and the diagnostic test are the same. For example, blood glucose test can be used as a screening test if it is given to someone who does not have any symptoms of diabetes. If the same test is given to someone with symptoms of diabetes to confirm a diagnosis of diabetes, it would be considered a diagnostic test.

The Natural History of Disease Progression

Below is a classic diagram of the course of a disease in an individual over time. At each point on the continuum, the degree to which intervention can be effective is dependent upon the type of disease. Similarly, the speed of progression from healthy to the final stage varies a lot by disease as well as an individual's characteristics.

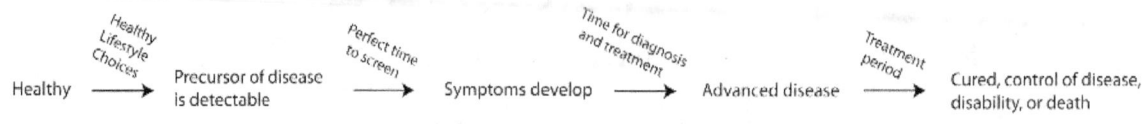

Natural history of disease progression

Screening occurs in two places on the continuum. The best time to screen is during the stage immediately prior to disease onset. For example, colonoscopy can detect polyps in the colon. Polyps are not cancer and if removed prevent cancer at that site. The second place screening occurs is when either the precursor of the disease is detectable or when symptoms develop. For example, a blood pressure screen can determine hypertension, a potential precursor to stoke. Another example is breast cancer screening to catches the disease is the earliest stage. Diagnosis in early stage dramatically improves survival. Although everyone agrees that reduction in morbidity and mortality is an important public health goal, there are several factors that need to be taken into consideration when deciding about implementing a screening program.

Population Screening Criteria

Four criteria for population based screening were proposed by Wilson and Jungner in a report to the World Health Organization more than 30 years ago. These are still considered relevant today.

1. Knowledge of the disease.

The prevalence of the disease must be balanced with the severity of the disease and the likelihood of effectiveness of treatment.

PKU Example

In 1934 a Norwegian doctor, Asbjorn Folling, discovered PKU (phenylketonuria) as the cause of severe mental retardation in 2 young children. PKU is called an error of metabolism because children cannot break down phenylalanine, an amino acid making up approximately 5% of all protein foods. Dr. Folling showed that PKU was an inherited disease. At that time, the prevalence of PKU in institutions for severely mentally retarded individuals in western counties was 1-2%. Blood tests were developed in the early 1960s to test for this genetic abnormality since, if caught early–within the first 2 weeks of life–mental retardation can often be prevented. In the United States, the newborn screening test for PKU is mandated by law in all states except Maryland and Wyoming.

This newborn screening test is worth the societal burden since the consequences of the disease are quite severe and early treatment is beneficial.

2. Feasibility of screening procedures.

Not only does the test need to be appropriate for disease identification, but patients have to agree to be tested. A classic example of a test that does not have wide acceptance is the fecal occult blood test for colorectal cancer.

3. Diagnosis and treatment.

A screening test can identify those at risk of the disease, in an early stage or precursor stage of the disease. This kind of screening, as opposed to diagnostic screen, has limited value if no treatment is available.

For example, someone diagnosed with pancreatic cancer has a very poor prognosis, typically 3 months to live. The early diagnosis will not change the prognosis of the disease since the cause of pancreatic cancer is unknown. In other words, precursors to pancreatic cancer are also unknown. Consequently, instituting a population-based screening program for this rare disease would not make sense.

4. Cost considerations

One misunderstanding is that screening programs always save money. However, this is not always true. If the disease is rare and the cost for the screening is high, there may be considerable health care costs to implement a national screening program. The cost consideration is one of the arguments used by some to resist implementing a national program for colonoscopy screening for colorectal cancer.

In the United States, cervical cancer, breast cancer, prostate cancer, colon cancer, diabetes and hypertension are diseases in which screening has been recommended with various degrees of compliance.

Case Studies

Prostate Cancer: PSA (prostate specific antigen) Screening Controversy

Prostate cells put out a small amount of protein, called prostatic specific antigen (PSA) that may be detected using a blood test. Since the amount of prostate tissue increases with age, PSA levels normally increase with age, so the normal range gradually increases from under 2.5 ng/ml between the ages of 40 and 49 to as high as 6.5 ng/ml by the age of 79.

It is common knowledge in the medical world that if you are male and live long enough, you are likely to have cancerous tissue in your prostate. It is also true that males are more likely to die *with* prostate cancer than to die *from* it. Therein lies the controversy. According to the Centers for Disease Control and Prevention (CDC), the current prostate specific antigen (PSA) test approved in 1986 by the Food and Drug Administration to screen for prostate cancer can detect the disease in its early stages. However, epidemiologic evidence is mixed and inconclusive about whether early detection actually saves lives because researchers do not know how quickly prostate cancer cells grow. Almost all older men have some prostate cancer cells at the time of their death. This may suggest that prostate cancer cells grow slowly. It is not clear whether the benefits of screening outweigh the risks of follow-up testing and cancer treatments.

People who support routine PSA screening for men over 45 years of age point out that it improves early diagnosis of a common, curable cancer at an earlier stage than can be detected by physical exam. Those who oppose routine screening state that it is costly and will result in unnecessary, invasive biopsies and treatment of people whose prostate problems would not have resulted in significant disease. Opponents to the PSA test also say the results often prompt men to undergo surgery or other treatments that leave them impotent or incontinent (impotent means inability to sustain an erection sufficient for sexual activity and incontinent means not having control over urination), even when there is little chance prostate cancer will kill them.

Breast Cancer: Mammography Screening Controversy

Mammograms are heavily promoted as a breast cancer prevention tool. Of all types of breast cancer, one type, called *in situ,* has increased from 2-3% in the early '80s to around 16% in the early '00 of all breast cancer diagnosis. Typically, the treatment is a lumpectomy (removal of the lump). In northern Europe, women diagnosed with *in situ* breast cancer who have it surgically removed are considered cured. Increased mammography use is the reason why the percent of *in situ* breast cancer has increased over time.

The controversy arises regarding the age at which women should be screened for breast cancer using a mammogram. Mainstream organizations, such as the American Cancer Society, the American College of Radiology and the National Cancer Advisory Board, part of the National Cancer Institute, recommend that women begin screening at age 40. However, epidemiology studies have not found consistent benefit of screening mammography before the age of 50 years.

Advocates for screening beginning at age 40 feel that this screening tool saves lives since many doctors believe that mammograms can detect a tumor 80% of the time. Those opposed to mammogram use before the age of 50 believe that the screen itself, an X-ray of the breast, puts women at an increased risk due to exposure to ionizing radiation, even though it is at a low dose. (Ionizing radiation is considered a risk factor for breast cancer.) Those who support mammogram use, argue that the dose is so low as to be of little concern. Another argument by those who support early use of mammograms is the type of breast cancer that is more common in younger women—a fast growing, aggressive cancer would be detected earlier through annual mammogram screening. Finally, critics of mammograms for younger women have emphasized the greater difficulty in detecting small tumors, which is the major reason for getting a mammogram, due to the denser breast tissue of young women.

As noted in the two case studies above screening is not without controversy. When a screening program in instituted, several bias need to be considered when evaluating the efficacy of the program.

Screening is the principle tool for secondary prevention. Implementing a screening program is not necessarily straightforward since the costs or burdens to the population need to weigh against the benefits. Even when a screening test has been developed, the quality of the test results needs to be considered. Usually changing patterns of screening directly influence the respective disease trends. The development of better screening tests will motivate some researchers in the quest to improve health for the populace.

Summary

Screening allows for the early detection of a disease. In most, but not all, cases, early detection leads to better health outcome. People diagnosed with an earlier stage of disease, often live longer. Screening is different from diagnosis, although the same test might be used. A diagnostic test confirms the disease.

Concept Reinforcement

1. What factors do you think are most important in deciding whether or not there should be a recommended screening test that is paid for by insurance? For example, do you think cost should be considered when deciding?

2. Why is there confusion between screening and diagnosis?

3. Do you think PSA should be given to every adult male over 45 years old? Why or why not.

Chapter 14 - Prevalence and Incidence

Chapter Objectives

- Define prevalence
- Define incidence
- Compare prevalence, incidence, and frequency

From birth to death, people experience many health states with varying frequency. Frequency means how often something happens. We all know stories of a seemingly perfectly healthy young person who suddenly and unexpectedly died one day. Although this often gets the most press, it is a very rare occurrence. The majority of people fluctuate from healthy, to sick, to be cured of that sickness—experiencing some disability—maintaining at a diminished level of health, to deceased. These states of health are dynamic in a population. At any one time, some of the population will be experiencing each of these states.

The most common measure is to count the number of cases of disease or health outcome. However, for a count to be descriptive of a group, it is expressed as a proportion. Proportions are often expressed as percentages by using the multiplier of 100. One of the central tasks in epidemiology is to determine the appropriate denominator to meaningfully describe and compare groups. The denominator must be the total number of people at risk for the disease. For highly contagious and deadly cases, such as anthrax, a single case will be front page news.

Another very common measure is rate. The difference between proportion and rate is that a rate involves a measure of time. The numerator is the frequency of the disease over a specific period of time and the denominator is a population, often at midpoint in the specific period. Another characteristic of a rate is that the denominator must be drawn from the case population. For example if we report the annual rate of birth defects, the numerator is the number of birth defects in a year and the denominator is the number of births in the same year.

In determining the frequency of disease, different denominators are chosen depending on the research goal and availability of data. For example, if a researcher is studying a disease frequency within a general population, the denominator will be different than if a research is studying the frequency of a disease (stroke, for example) in a population of people with hypertension. Paying attention to the denominator is a skill that an epidemiologist improves with practice.

Prevalence

Prevalence, sometimes known as point prevalence, means the number of people in the population of interest (e.g., school district, city, county, state) who have the particular disease or illness at a point in time, usually when the survey is administered. For example, if there are 5 people with the disease outcome of interest in a population of 200, prevalence is 2.5%. Prevalence measures are proportions. Although prevalence is often described as a rate, it is not. Remember that a rate has a time dimension and prevalence does not.

Prevalence tells us nothing about how long someone has had the disease—it could be a day, a year or many years. Some people like to think of prevalence as a snap shot in time that tells us the number of people with the disease.

Prevalence is useful to measure the burden of disease in the community. For example, how many people with uncontrolled asthma live in the community? This prevalence number will help determine the number of clinics, the need for emergency medical services, the number and type of health care providers, etc. Prevalence numbers are very useful in planning health services.

Case Studies of Prevalence Data

The following are case studies the shows the usefulness of prevalence data.

Prevalence of Swallowing Disorders

Researchers were interested in determining whether swallowing disorders, such as difficulty eating due to some problem swallowing, was an issue for hospital patients. The researchers counted the number of patients with swallowing disorders over a 3-week period in two hospitals and reported that 13% of the patients had swallowing disorders. This prevalence was much higher than they had anticipated and they ended their article by calling for resources to be used to deal with this problem.

Celiac Disease and Patients with Type 1 Diabetes

Celiac disease: An autoimmune disease which disrupts absorption of nutrients in the small intestine. Gluten has been identified as a trigger.

Type 1 Diabetes, also known as childhood diabetes, is disease in which the pancreas does not make insulin. Insulin is a hormone that helps glucose get into cells to give a person energy.

If a physician is aware of a high prevalence of celiac disease in patients with type 1 diabetes, s/he might be more likely to ask the patient about specific symptoms and/or order a test for celiac disease.

Incidence Rate

Now we are going to turn our attention to incidence rate. Incidence data is a fundamental measure used for research on the causes of disease. Disease frequency can be measured using prevalence or incidence. Incidence refers to *new* cases in a population at risk during a specific time period whereas prevalence is a snapshot of all individuals with the disease without a time dimension. For prevalence, some of these individuals may have had the disease for years and some may have been diagnosed in the previous month. In contrast, for incidence, the numerator is the frequency of new cases which means people with a history of the disease are not included in the numerator.

The denominator is the number of persons at risk for developing the disease during that period of time. Unlike mortality data, in which everyone has some probability of dying, some individuals do not have a chance of diagnosis for some diseases/illnesses. For example, to calculate the incidence of ovarian cancer, women who have had an oophorectomy (both ovaries removed) would be excluded from the denominator as well as men, obviously. For infectious diseases, those who have lifetime immunity against recurrence would be excluded from the denominator.

For example, 75 adults in a town of 25,000 adults have been diagnosed with celiac disease in 2009. The incidence is 75 divided by 25,000 equals 0.003. It we want to express the incidence rate per 1000 adults, then we multiply by 1000. The incidence rate is 3 per 1000 adults. Reporting the data as 3 per 1000 persons is more understandable to the general population than stating the incidence as 0.003.

Connection Between Prevalence and Incidence

The interrelationship between prevalence and incidence is as follows: prevalence of a disease is proportional to the incidence rate multiplied by (average) duration of the disease. Consequently, for diseases of short duration and high incidence, the prevalence is similar to the incidence. Why is that? For a disease of short duration, either the patients recover their health or die. Therefore, over time the number of people with a history of the disease in the population is virtually zero because those who had the disease eventually die from some other cause. Remember, incidence does not take into consideration those with a history of a disease since the numerator only contains new cases. Some infectious diseases meet these criteria. In contrast, many chronic diseases have low incidence and long duration. With this scenario, as time passes, the number of people living with the disease increases so that at any one time period the prevalence would be higher than the incidence.

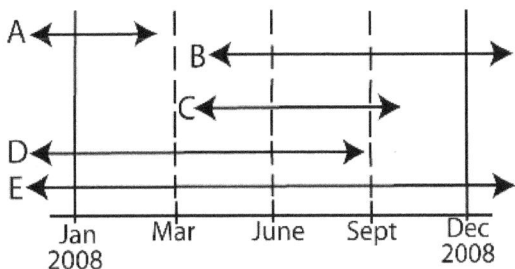

Example of persons A, B, C, D, E and their respective duration of disease in 2008

In the above figure, we are going to ignore the denominator. For 2008, there were 2 incidences of the disease, person B and C. For the other persons, their disease began before 2008 so there was only 2 new cases of the disease. In June of 2008, the prevalence of the disease was 4 cases. At that point in time, there was 4 people with the disease. Only person A did not have the disease at that time.

Summary

Two measures in epidemiology is prevalence and incidence. Prevalence measures the proportion of cases in the population at risk. In contrast, incidence measures the number of new cases in the population at risk over a specific period of time. For both of these measures, it is important to pay close attention to determining the population at risk for the denominator.

Concept Reinforcement

1. Why is prevalence an important measure for population health studies?

2. What would be the formula to calculate the prevalence of females in the class right now? (Hint: what is the numerator and what is the denominator?)

3. What does incidence tell us that is different from prevalence?

Chapter 15 - Ethics

Chapter Objectives

- Describe the Tuskegee study and Nazi human experimentations
- Describe the 3 criteria for ethical research
- List the elements of consent

Nazi Experiments During WWII

During WWII, medical experiments were conducted on large number of concentration camp prisoners. The prisoners were forced to participate in these experiments. They did not volunteer. They did not consent to be part of the experiments. For example, in one experiment prisoners were forced to float in a tank of ice water for up to 5 hours. The Nazis were using prisoners to figure out different ways of rewarming survivors. At the end of the war, doctors captured by Allied forces were put on trial. One of the results of the trial was the writing of the Nuremberg Code in 1946. This code calls for voluntary consent of participants, avoidance of unnecessary pain and suffering, and a belief that the experiment will not end in death or disability.

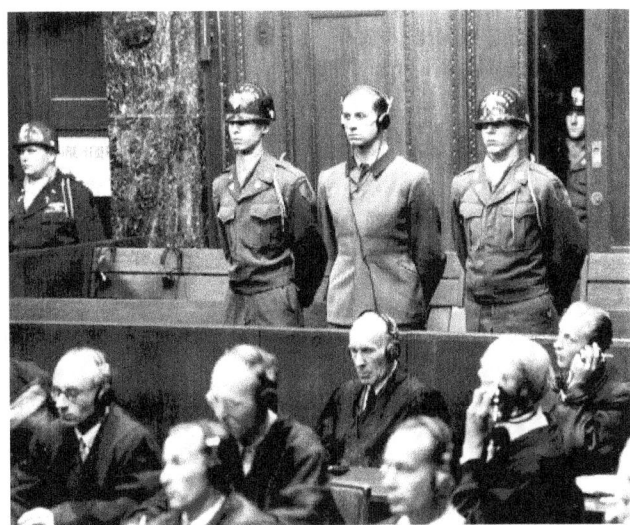

Death by hanging is pronounced by a U.S. War Crimes Tribunal at Nuremberg upon Adolf Hitler's personal physician, 43-year old Karl Brandt. Brandt, who was also Hitler's Reich Commissar for Health and Sanitation, was indicted by U.S. prosecutors, along with 22 other Nazi doctors and SS officers, on war crimes charges. This was the first case of alleged criminals being tried after the judgment of the International Military Tribunal. The Tribunal found him guilty on all four counts, charging him with conspiracy in aggressive wars, war crimes, crimes against humanity, and membership in the criminal SS organization. Among those criminal acts, was his participation in and consent to using concentration camp inmates as guinea pigs in horrible medical experiments, supposedly for the benefit of the armed forces.

He was hanged at Landsberg prison on June 2, 1948 because of his execution of thousands of helpless political, racial, and religious persecutees. This occurred after U.S. Military Commander Gen. Lucius D. Clay and the U.S. Supreme court upheld the Nuremberg Tribunal's judgment. In a long-winded speech that was finally muffled when the black hood was thrown over his head, Brandt shouted arrogantly, "It is no shame to stand on this scaffold; I have served my country as have others before me."

Hitler was also imprisoned in this fortress-like building near Munich in 1923 following his unsuccessful Munich putsch. During his confinement, he wrote what was later to become the Nazi bible, "Mein Kampf."

Image courtesy of the US Army. Caption modified from the Telford Taylor Papers, held by Columbia University Law School.

The Tuskegee Syphilis Study (1932-1972)

A study of untreated syphilis in rural impoverished African American males was conducted in Macon County, Alabama from 1932 to 1972. Volunteers from the community responded to an announcement of the study and 400 men with syphilis and 200 men without syphilis were enrolled. One important aim of the study was to determine the prevalence and severity of syphilitic disease process. The men were told the doctors were studying "bad blood." Various methods were used to maintain and stimulate study participants' interest. Free medicines, burial assistance or insurance, free hot meals on the days of examination, transportation to and from the hospital, and an opportunity to stop in town on the return trip to shop or visit with their friends on the streets all helped. Through the tireless efforts of the project nurse, a very high number of participants remained in the study (87%). At the start of the study, there was no proven treatment for syphilis. However, even after penicillin became a standard cure for the disease in 1947, the medicine was withheld from the men. The Tuskegee scientists wanted to continue to study how the disease spreads and kills. The experiment lasted four decades, until public health workers leaked the story to the media. This medical study parallels the medical experiments on WW II prisoners of war in its level of unethical behavior.

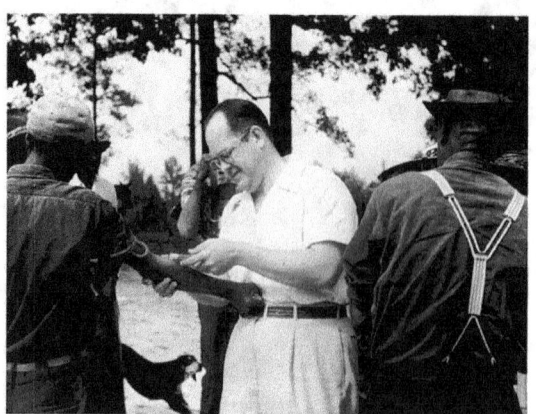

Examination, Tuskegee Study

Image courtesy of the National Archives and Records Administration

Willowbrook Hepatitis Study (1963-1966)

Research studies took place at a New York state supported institution called Willowbrook State School. This was an institution in which mentally disabled children were admitted. The research study was designed to gain an understanding of the natural history of infectious hepatitis. The children at the institution were infected with the hepatitis virus. During the 3 years of the study, Willowbrook did not allow any new admissions. However, the study was able to admit new patients to the institution since it had its own space. Thus, in some cases, parents could admit their child to Willowbrook only if they agreed to have their child participant in this study. Many felt that the children and parents had little choice in participating in the study.

Belmont Report

A meeting in the late 70s was held to address problems arising from researchers acting in questionable ways. The Nazi experiments, the Tuskegee Syphilis Study, the Willowbrook Hepatitis Study and the Tearoom Trade study are examples of some questionable ethics. The Belmont report is an important document. It was written in 1979. The name of the report comes from the Belmont Conference Center where the report was drafted. The Belmont report explains the ethical principles underlying the medical research in a clear and concise way.

There are three fundamental ethical principles for using human subjects for research.

1. Respect for persons. This means the researchers need to treat participants with respect and courtesy. Participation in the study occurs with informed consent by the participants. The wishes and decision-making ability of the participants must be respected.

2. Beneficence. This means that the research must maximize benefits for the research project while minimizing risks to the research subjects

3. Justice. This means that the research is fairly administered. The costs and benefits to the potential research participants are fairly distributed. The researchers do not exploit potential participants. The fairness principle goes both ways—fairness in terms of who is included and excluded in a research study and fairness in terms of who benefits from the research and who bears its burdens.

The Belmont report serves as a historical document. It provides the moral framework for using humans in research. It is also the basis of the federal regulations regarding the use of humans in research.

Informed Consent

One important element of participating in a research study is informed consent. Informed consent means that the person has a clear understanding of the risks and benefits of participating in the study. Consenting can occur in two distinct ways. A person can give active consent. This generally means a signed consent form. A person's action can imply consent. If a person fills out a questionnaire, this is implied consent. For a participant who did not want to participate in the study, s/he just would not fill out the questionnaire. The same concept applies if a researcher calls you on the telephone and explains a study. This person will ask you if you would be willing to answer some question. If you say yes and answer some questions, this is an example of implied consent.

Elements of Consent

There are many required elements of consent. An 8th grade reading level is the target for this letter. The language of each of the points below has to be at the 8th grade level and appropriate for the people who are potential participants.

Below is a list of eight common elements that are included in a consent letter.

1. A statement that the study involves research. An explanation of the purposes of the research and expected duration.

2. A description of the procedures to be followed, and identification of any procedures which are experimental.

3. A description of any reasonably foreseeable risks or discomforts to the subject.

4. A description of any benefits to the subject or others which may be reasonably expected from the research

5. A disclosure of appropriate alternative procedures or courses of treatment, if any, that might be advantageous to the subject

6. A statement describing the extent, if any, to which confidentiality of records identifying the subject will be maintained. For research involving more than minimal risk, an explanation as to whether any compensation and an explanation as to whether any medical treatments are available if injury occurs

7. An explanation of whom to contact for answers

8. A statement that participation is voluntary

It is easy to see why the consent letter is long. All of these elements must be in the consent letter.

Summary

Historically, epidemiologist did not have any oversight. They could do whatever research they wanted to do. In a few situations, this lead to a clear violation of human rights. In the largest violation that took place during WWII, some of the Nazi researchers were put on trial for war crimes. In other situations, no criminal action was taken against the researcher. Due to some of these questionable practices, studies by researchers in the United States are examined carefully by peers and institutions review boards to make sure that human rights are maintained.

Concept Reinforcement

1. What was unethical about the Tuskegee Syphilis Study?

2. What was unethical about the Willowbrook Hepatitis Study?

3. Consent letters are typically long and detailed since elements of consent are required. Do you think any of the elements of consent could be deleted from the letter?

Chapter 16 - Risk Factors

Chapter Objectives

- Describe age and sex as risk factors
- List the issues regarding the use of race
- Describe the components necessary for occupational coding

Although people differ from one another in an infinite number of ways, there are common characteristics that are important to consider in epidemiology. These characteristics are described below and include age, sex, race, ethnicity, income, education and occupation. Many of these characteristics can be found on the census. Every 10 years the US population is counted. The sole purpose of the censuses is to obtain general information about the population. It began in 1790 and continues today.

Age

The single most important personal characteristic in health research is age. The first step in an epidemiologic study is to look at the ages of the population under study. This alone might be the determining factor that describes the population's health risk. Most chronic diseases are age-related meaning that the older a person gets the higher the risk of being diagnosed with a chronic disease.

Fortunately, age is one of the easiest pieces of information to obtain in the Unites States. The U.S census provided age-related population data at various levels of geographic units. In addition, age is a commonly collected item on many surveys.

Sex

Similar to age, sex is generally collected. Knowing if a participant is male or female sometimes is important. In general, women tend to have more diseases and illnesses and men tend to die younger. The reason for this general trend is not clear. It may be due to biological differences between the sexes or it may be due to differences in life experiences. In any case, it is often useful to collect this information.

Race and Ethnicity

Race reflects a social definition. It is unique for each country. For example, in the 2000 U.S. census, individual could select multiple categories when asked to self-identify their own race. A few diseases are more common in some racial groups, such as sickle cell anemia in Blacks and breast cancer in Ashkenazi Jewish populations from Northern Europe. However, similar to sex, striking differences can be noted in disease incidence, severity and death rate among the races. The reason for these differences is unknown and may reflect biological differences or differences in life experiences

Ethnicity is based on culture. Ethnicity is different from race. Ethnicity can be divided into 2 categories: "Hispanic or Latino/Latina" versus "Not Hispanic or Latino/Latina." Hispanic or Latino/Latina is defined by the U.S. Census as a person of Cuban, Mexican, Puerto Rican, South or Central American or other Spanish culture or origin regardless of race.

However, using race and ethnicity data can be problematic. Studies ask about race and ethnicity differently. When this happens, making comparison between studies is very difficult. In addition, race and ethnicity definition have changed over time.

United States Census Race Categories in Selected Years from 1860-2000				
1860	1870	1900	1970	2000
White	White	White	White	White[1]
Black	Black	Black (of Negro descent)	Black or Negro	Black, African American, or Negro[2]
Quadroon*	Quadroon*			
	Chinese	Chinese	Chinese	Chinese
	Indian	Indian	Indian (American)	American Indian or Native American[3]
	Japanese	Japanese	Japanese	Japanese
			Filipino	Filipino
				Asian Indian[4]
			Korean	Korean
			Hawaiian	Native Hawaiian[5]
				Vietnamese Guamanian or Chamorro
				Samoan
				Other Asian
				Other Pacific Islander
				Some other race

Source: 200 Years of U.S. Census Taking: Population and Housing Questions 1790-1990. U.S. Department of Commerce. U.S. Bureau of the Census

*In 1890, mulatto was defined as a person who was 3/8th to 5/8th black. A quadroon was 1/4th black and an octoroon was 1/8th black.

[1] Persons having origins in any of the original peoples of Europe, the Middle East or North Africa

[2] A person having origins in any of the black racial groups of Africa. Terms such as "Haitian" or "Negro" can be used in addition to "Black or African American"

[3] A person have origins in any of the original people of North or South America (including Central America) and who maintain tribal affiliation or community attachment

[4] A person having origins in any of the original people of the Far East, Southeast Asia of the Indian subcontinent including for example, Cambodia, China, India, Japan, Korea, Malaysia, Pakistan, the Philippine Islands, Thailand and Vietnam

[5] A person having origins in any of the original peoples of Hawaii, Guam, Samoa, or other Pacific Islands

Socioeconomic Status

Socioeconomic status (SES) is a characteristic made up of many pieces. However, in the majority of studies, education, income and/or occupation are used for SES status. Participants usually do not have a problem answering the question about their education level. In contrast, income is less clear cut. Sometimes people are uncomfortable answering a question about their income. In addition, when asking about income, a person could respond with his or her own income or the income of the family (aka: household income) or some combination. Further, individual may not think about all sources of income but rather just report on their weekly or monthly paycheck amount.

Occupations

People change careers about 3 times in their lifetime. Career is different than occupation or job. A career is a combination and series of occupational positions held during the course of a lifetime. That means that the series of jobs has something in common. In contrast, a job is a position held with specific duties with an employer. When asking about occupation, some researchers ask for the first job ever held that was at least 30 hours a week for at least 6 months. Some ask for current job. However, most ask for the "most representative job" held over one's lifetime. Unlike asking about education or income, to use the data collected on occupation, it has to be coded.

Coding Data

To analyze data and produce study results all information collected has to be turned into numbers. Some data are given as numbers, such as age. Other data are not given as numbers and these data needed to be coded. In other words, these data need to have numbers assigned. As a simple illustration, if someone checked 'yes' to the question about having a tetanus vaccine, this '√' could not be analyzed. Rather, the answer to this question will be coded as "yes" = 1 and "no" = 2 and for those who didn't answer this question = 3. Therefore, all participants would be coded as 1, 2, or 3 for the answer to this question. These numbers *can* then analyzed.

Occupational Elements

For occupational jobs to be coded three pieces of information are needed: industry, job title and duties. Identifying the industry and job title is straightforward. This very simple question about duties, however, is very important for coding purposes. Although the question may seem unnecessary in some cases, the response often permits more accurate coding of the occupation. Obtaining detailed information on the job duties will help with coding. For example, in the telecommunication industry, telephone company serviceman is the job title. The duties could be installs telephone in the home (this would be given one code) versus repairs telephone transmission lines (this would be given an entirely different code).) Once the data have been collected, the coding can be done using an online reference, such as One*Net.

Summary

It is important to collect all the necessary information about the participants. Most studies collect age, sex, race, education and income. Depending on the study, occupational information will also be collected. In all cases, the data collected needs to be coded in such a way that the information can be analyzed.

Concept Reinforcement

1. What would be other information that participants in a study may be reluctant to provide?

2. Census data is used in numerous way including epidemiological studies. Although people are "required" to fill out a census form, some people do not. Should people who do not fill out a census survey be fined? Explain.

3. If you had to create an indicator variable that identified people of different socio-economic status, what information would you want?

Chapter 17 - Sample, Population, and Sample Size

Chapter Objectives

- Define a sample
- Define a population
- Compare sample vs. population

Most health research collects data from individuals. Paradoxically, researchers often want to know intimate details about individuals but researchers are not interested in actually knowing the individual. Individual data are stripped of identifying information and compiled into a dataset. These data are used to tell a story about the group under study.

> **Paradox**
> something that seems to contradict itself, even though it is true.

Two terms in statistics are important to know the difference: population and sample.

A population means ALL individuals. A sample is a subset of the population. The analogy is a whole pie is the population and a piece of the pie is the sample. The sample is taken from the population of interest. To continue the analogy, if we are interested I figuring out the average number of cherries in a cherry pie, we do not want to sample any kind of pie. We want to sample cherry pies. The other piece of information to realize is that population means ALL members. For cherry pies, it would be an impossible task to collect every single cherry pie in the world. Therefore, we would have to gather a sample of cherry pies.

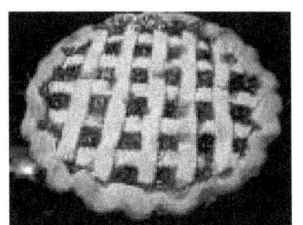

Cherry pie

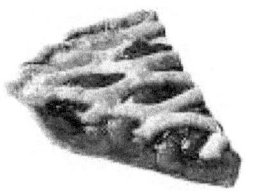

Piece of cherry pie

To illustrate the difference between sample and population, let's look at driving as our topic. The researcher is interested in figuring out the predictors of motor vehicle crashes in California in 2010 data. The researcher defines a crash as having a police accident report filed. The population would be all motor vehicle crash reports in 2010. If there are electronic records of these reports AND the electronic records are sent to a central location, the researcher could use the population of vehicle crashes in 2010 to determine the predictors of a crash. However, if the police reports were not enter electronically or were not sent to a central location, it would be virtually impossible for the researcher to compile all the police reports. In the second case, the researcher would use a sample of motor vehicle crash reports for the study. There are standard ways to take a sample from a population. For the purposes of this chapter, the important point is to understand the difference between sample and population.

Sample Size

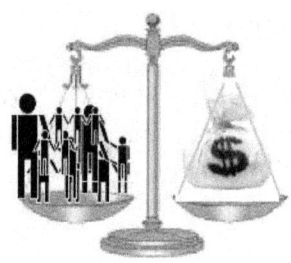

Scale balances sample size and study cost

How big does a sample need to be? The bigger the sample size, the smaller the random error and the higher likelihood of finding an effect. However, the bigger the sample size, the more expensive (and possibly more time consuming) the study. Researchers weigh these two competing interests: reduction of random error though increased number of participants and cost of the project.

If a sample is too small, in other words, too few people are enrolled in the project, the researcher will run into one of two problems. S/he may fail to find any meaningful result and/or the researcher will not be able to generalize his/her research findings.

If the samples size is too big, there are three issues. The first issue is a waste of resources since the researcher need not have gathered all that data. Remember for most cases, gathering data costs money. A second issue is a waste of respondents' time since some of their data were not needed. The study results would have been the same with a fewer number of participants. The third problem is that a very large study has the power to find significant results for very small, even clinically inconsequential differences.

For public opinion polls, such as the Gallup Poll that is done during election years to give the public an idea of how the presidential candidates are doing, the rule of thumb is 1500 randomly selected people is enough to provide the estimate of the whole population's opinion on a subject. More than 1500, will not improve the estimate.

When figuring out how many people to survey, the researcher realizes that as the population size increases, the percentage of people needed to achieve a high level of accuracy decrease rapidly. In other words, to obtain the same level of confidence in the study results, for larger population the researcher would need a smaller percentage of people surveyed and for a smaller population the researcher would need a larger percentage of people surveyed.

Summary

Everyone makes generalizations about the world through sampling. For example, we might select a book to purchase by reading a few pages. Often in the fruit section of the grocery story, we either visually inspect the stand of fruit or pinch a few fruit to select the best one. However, researchers have clear rules to decide on whether they can takes use a population or need to take a sample to answer their questions. If they need to take a sample, they pay special attention to figuring out how many samples are needed to answer their questions.

Concept Reinforcement

1. What would be an example of a question that the population could be used to answer?

2. What would be an example of a slightly different question that only a sample could be used to answer?

3. What are two examples of sampling that you do in your daily life? A generalization will have been made through this sampling.

Chapter 18 - Sources of Data

Chapter Objectives

- List the key characteristics of any dataset
- List vital statistics mandated for collection
- Discuss the pros and cons of datasets

No matter what kind of study the researcher does, it is only as good as the quality of the data. Epidemiology deals with populations. One reason the study of populations is important is that the findings may be able to be generalized. Secondly, data on populations are needed to make estimates on the frequency of diseases, illnesses, injuries and deaths. To help researchers, federal agencies compile a great deal of information about the population. Much of this information is helpful to researches.

Dataset Characteristics

Several characteristics are any dataset must be described for the researcher to understand how it can be used to answer his/her research question(s).

Data Source

The first piece of information is finding out the source of the data. Are the data from physician's records, from survey of the general population, from vital statistics (birth or death records), from registry such as a statewide cancer registry? The source of the data is very important to know.

Availability of the Data

Some data are publicly available to anyone who signs a confidentiality agreement. Other data are less easily obtained. In other cases, some data will only be released to the researcher when any elements that could identify an individual are stripped from the records.

Collection Date

When the data was collected will matter greatly. The data collected before or after a public policy can have dramatic influence on the answers, the participants give to particular questions. For example, participants would answer the question about seat belt use much different before the mandatory seat belt in a state than after the law was enacted.

Sampling Plan

The plan used to collect the data is very important. This will tell the researcher about the usefulness of these data. If the data were collected from a very special population, it may not be very useful to the researcher. For example if a survey collected data about Hmong's dietary habits, this information would not be very useful if the researcher was studying eating habits of all people.

Data Dictionary

A data dictionary contains at least three elements to be useful: the variable, the question on the survey, the type of variable. Specifically, the exact questions that were asked of participants, the variable names associated to the questions and the variable type (numeric, character, or date) must be available for the researcher to be able to use these data. For example, in the dataset a variable is called "dob." However, the question could have been "What is your date of birth?" or "What is your first born child's date of birth?" Without having the questions, it would be impossible to know the meaning of the variable "dob."

Identifiable and De-identifiable Data

Data can be divided into two groups: data that contain personal identifiers and data that do not contain personal identifiers. Personal identifiers are variables in the dataset that can be used to identify a person. This is particularly important in epidemiology since protecting the confidentiality of a person is very important. Several variables can identify an individual alone or in combination. Some of these are name, social security number, address, any date (except year), telephone number, fax number, email address, and medical record number. These must be stripped from the record before the researcher has access to de-identifiable data. De-identifying data allows the participants identity to be protected.

For researchers who use identifiable data, they would NEVER publish any results so that anyone reading the article could identify a person. Often the federal and state governmental agencies use the rule of five. It means that if five or less people are grouped together, then that number is not published. For example, if there were less than five women diagnosed with breast cancer in 2008 in a rural county in Missouri, then on the table listing number of breast cancer cases by county would not show any data for this county. In some situations, a rule of 20 or 50 is used. This means that at least 20 or 50 people have to be in a group for the number to be shown.

Advantages and Disadvantages of Pre-existing Data

Probably the clearest advantage of using pre-existing data is that it is already collected. It is much cheaper for the researcher to use pre-existing data than to collect his/her own data. The biggest disadvantage of using pre-existing data is that it rarely contains all the information that the researcher wishes was obtained. Sometimes the data were collected for some other reason besides a health query. In this case, many of the standard items in a survey such as age and sex of the respondent might not have been asked.

The data in any study has its own particular strengths and weaknesses. For example, a birth registry that contains information from the birth certificates is pretty complete. This means that almost all births would be recorded in the registry. In contrast, some of the elements on the birth certificate are not trustworthy, such as the baby's race. In this case, the baby's race may be recorded based on the mother's skin color or the mother's last name.

Vital Statistics

The government mandates the collection of certain vital statistics on everyone in the country. These statistics include birth, death, marriage and divorce information. These records are maintained for every person in the country. Every child who is born receives a birth certificate, which details the names of the parents, the date of birth, and the place of birth. Likewise, a death certificate is issued for every person who dies. This information is essential for maintaining population records, as well as dealing with the legal issues surrounding birth and death. Marriage status is also considered a vital statistics. Both marriages and divorces are recorded as part of the vital statistics of a population.

Summary

Primary data is data that the researcher collects from participants whereas secondary data is data that has already been collected by someone else. In both cases, the quality of the data is important. High quality data translates into the ability to have more confidence in the study results. Sometimes secondary is available but in other cases the researcher needs to collect his/her own data to answer a specific question. Vital statistics include birth, death, marriage and divorce information.

Concept reinforcement

1. What is particularly important about data collected by federal agencies, such as the census?

2. Why is it important hide the number of people who have a particular disease if it is less than 5?

3. What kind of data would you prefer to use, primary or secondary?

Chapter 19 - Types of Surveys and Variables

Chapter Objectives

- Describe the four types of survey data collection
- Define validity
- Define reliability

A survey is one way of gathering information from study participants. The survey must have an objective. An objective is a question that can be answered from the responses to the survey. The best question to ask yourself when you are designing a survey is "What do I really want to know?" This is also a good question to ask when you review each question in the survey. A health survey, which is what epidemiologists do, asks people about health issues. A health survey can be used in all kinds of study designs. There are four common ways to collect data: through the mail, by telephone, in person, and using the internet. In designing a questionnaire, there is always a tradeoff between asking too many question that are not necessary to answer the question and too few questions.

Mailed Surveys

For success, researchers need an accurate mailing address. If participants are not happy with the design or the topic, they will be less likely to complete the survey.

Telephone Interviews

Telephone interviewers often enter the data into the computer as it is being obtained from the respondent. Of course, the researcher needs to have a telephone number to call the participants. Finding a person's telephone number is becoming more difficult with the popularity of cell phones. Similar to the mailed survey, if the participants are not immediately engaged, it is likely they will hang up or not even pick up the telephone.

In-person Data Collection

The interviewer has a laptop computer, asks questions to the participant, and enters the data as the respondent answers the questions. This is called CAPI, computer assistant personal interviewing. Another method for in-person interviewing is to video or tape record the interview. In both of these situations, the material will have to be transcribed. The final situation is where the study personnel hands out a survey and waits while the participant fills it out and returns it to the study personnel.

> **Transcribe**
> To transfer information from an audio or video record to paper records.

Web-based Data Collection

Although appealing, the number of people who respond is typically low. Web based surveys can only be used for those who have computers or who have access to computer.

Variables

A variable is the name used to analyze the data. In an analytical program, a question is turned into a variable name. The answer options are the values that populate the variable. For example, "How old are you?" become an "age" variable. The values will be from 1-110 or whatever the age range of the participants. There are three types of variables: number, text, and date. All questions can be reduced to these three types of variables.

Number

A number variable can be either a whole number (e.g., 1, 2, 3) or an integer (e.g., 1.2, 3.8). Whether the participant responds to a question by using the whole number or integer depends on how the question was asked.

A question such as "What is your GPA?" requires an integer response. In contrast, "How many children do you have?" requires a whole number response.

In analytical programs, if any part of an answer is not a number, then the variable becomes a text variable. For example, if a respondents telephone number is given as 573-493-2332, then the variable becomes a text variable. In contrast, if the telephone number is entered as 5734932332, then the variable can be a number.

Date

A data variable provides day, month and year. Sometimes only month and year are provided. In analytical programs, the data variable is converted to some number by the program. Typically, the statistician does not know the formula used in the calculation and it really does not matter. The only important point is that the date be entered in the same way. This means that it can be entered as numbers (e.g., 4/4/10) or as text and numbers (e.g., April 4, 2010). As long as the dates are entered in the same way for any questions, there will be no problems.

Character

The third type of variable is a character. Just as the name implies, a character variable contains at least one symbol or letter of the alphabet. The concern with character fields is that the spacing, spelling and capitalization have to be identical in all entries for the answers to be counted properly. For example, if the answer to participant's city is St. Louis, the entry has to be St. Louis for everyone who lives there. Otherwise, counting the number of participants who live in St. Louis will give data on each spelling variation. St Louis is different from St. Louis. Similarly, St. louis is different from St. Louis. As you can see, there are numerous variations in this data entry. Consequently, when possible, researchers usually recode text fields to numbers. An answer to "Are you a) male or b) female?" will be entered as a 1 or 2 in the database. The number 1 means a male response and a number 2 means a female response.

Data Validity and Reliability

Data validity and reliability are two ways researchers assess the quality of the research conducted. Data validity is generally considered the correctness and reasonableness of the data. The question to ask here is whether the data collected during the survey actual reflect what is happening. Data reliability is a measure of reproducibility of the data. For example, if you ask the same person a question that has only one correct answer, such as birth date, on five different occasions and you get the same answer five times, the data are reliable. However, if the person gives different answers, the data are probably not reliable. It is possible for data to be highly reliable, but invalid. In other words, it is possible to do something the same way many times and get the same result. However, if the tool you are using introduces bias to the data, all of the data could be incorrect even though they are reliable.

Summary

Using surveys is one of the key ways that epidemiologists collect information in their quest to understand risk factors associated with health outcomes. Each question in a survey is turned into a variable. How old are you? becomes an age variable. The three common variables are numbers, characters or dates. By thoughtful collection of information, epidemiologists can answer questions about risk factors and health.

Concept Reinforcement

1. What are the benefits of asking as many questions as a researcher as possible? In other words, pages and pages of questions?

2. What are the disadvantages of asking as many questions as a researcher as possible? In other words, pages and pages of questions?

3. Do you think people would respond differently if asked "What is you're age versus What is your birthdate?" How about "How much do you make?" versus "Select the category that best matches your income?" Explain.

Chapter 20 - Constructing Survey Questions

Chapter Objectives

- Define the main properties of a good survey
- Identify features of a problematic question
- List six characteristics of a good question
- Describe the limitations of the three types of questions

A survey is one way of gathering information from study participants. The survey must have an objective. An objective is a question that can be answered from the responses to the survey. The best question to ask yourself when you are designing a survey is "What do I really want to know?" This is also a good question to ask when you review each question in the survey. A health survey, which is what epidemiologists do, asks people about health issues. A health survey can be used in all kinds of study designs.

One of the biggest misconceptions is that writing good survey questions is easy. Since we speak the language and we ask questions every day, we assume that we are all skilled at making up survey questions. In fact, few people can easily write good survey questions. In class, students have heated arguments with their teacher about a test because the question or the answer options were not clear. The benefit of classroom testing is that students have the opportunity to challenge the question one-on-one with the teacher. In surveys, this opportunity is not possible. Consequently, the questions need to be carefully written.

Important Points in Writing Survey Questions

Everyone needs to understand the answer options to multiple choice questions in exactly the same way. Answers to multiple choice questions must be stated clearly. It is very important to remember the participants to whom the questions are being asked. It is possible for different participants to understand the same choices differently if they are not carefully phrased.

Double Barreled Questions

Only one question is asked and answered per question—no "double barreled" questions. If a question seems too complex, it is important to make it simpler or split the complex question into two questions.

For example, Do you drive or take the bus everyday to school? Yes ( ) No ( )

A respondent can answer "yes" to "Do you drive?" and " No" to the part of the question that asks about taking the bus.

Mutually Exclusive Questions

The categories (answer options) must be mutually exclusive. Answers to multiple choice questions must not overlap in any way. This will lead to confusion among the respondents and likely bias the results of the data analysis.

For example, "What is your annual household income in 2009?"

    a. Less than $20,000

    b. $20,000–$50,000

    c. $50,000–$75,000

    d. $75,000–$100,000

    e. More than $100,000

If a respondent's household income is $50,000, which category does the respondent select, b or c? These answer choices are not mutually exclusive.

Continuous Data

The categories (answer options) that use continuous data include all possibilities within the range. Consider the nature of the question being asked and the standards used in the target population. For example, homes can have inside and outside bathrooms. They can also have full, half and quarter baths. If one is asking about bathrooms, it is important to offer all of the options so respondents can answer accurately.

For example "How many bathrooms are inside your home?"

    a. 1

    b. 2

    c. 3

    d. more than 3

What answer choice would the participant select for 1.5 bathrooms?

Unbias Questions

The questions must be unbiased, meaning the question or answer choices are stated objectively. They do not encourage the participants to answer one way or the other.

For example, "Which one of the following do you feel is *most* responsible for the increase in obesity in children?"

    a. fewer safe places to play outside

    b. bad food choices

    c. children watching too much television

    d. lack of physical exercise during the school day

The term "bad" in option b has a value connotation. A negative connotation as part of the answer option is not part the other choices. Option c also has a value connotation because the words "too much" are used.

Negative Questions

Avoid negative questions since respondents will often skip over the negative and answer the question as if it was worded in the positive. The human brain tends to ignore the word "don't." For example, if you ask a person about the last time they did not do something, they will likely respond with information on the last time they did that specific action.

Time Reference

Provide a time reference when appropriate. For example, it is important when asking about annual income to include a time frame so that data can be compared across all the respondents. One person may think of income in term of the calendar year (Jan-Dec) and others may think of it in terms of a fiscal year (some other 12 month period).

"How many international conferences did you attend?"

    a. Did not attend any conference

    b. 1 conference

    c. 2 conferences

    d. 3 conferences

There is no time reference so the participants might answer for one year or during their career.

Three General Mistakes in Writing Questions

Poor survey question development is the biggest mistake made in epidemiologic research; and it is even committed by experienced researchers.

Another mistake is that researchers want to ask many more questions than are necessary. As the survey gets longer, less respondents will take the time to complete the survey. Collecting too much information wastes the respondents' time since this extra information will rarely be used.

The third mistake that researchers make when constructing a survey is not doing their homework. This means that they do not read the literature thoroughly to find out what is known and what should be asked.

Types of Questions

Question types include open ended, multiple choice, and yes-no (also true-false)

Open-ended

Turning responses to an open ended question into data is very time-consuming. There is software to help with this but first the response has to be put into electronic format. After that specialize data analysis is performed to have qualitative information. Except for researchers that are interested in this type of data, open-ended questions are usually avoided in survey design.

Multiple Choice

Multiple choice questions provide several answer options that give the respondent a choice but, if not properly put together the quality of the survey. Many of these issues are described above.

Yes-No

Limited information is gained by asking yes-no questions or true-false questions. They are often used to select a population with a very specific characteristic for a section of a survey.

Summary

Gathering data from surveys is one of the fundamental tools of epidemiology. Being able to design a survey that effectively and efficiently gathers data to answer a focused question is a skill that develops with practice. Many researchers have experienced the dismay of either asking a poor question (and therefore not being able to use the data gathered for that questions) or not asking a vital question. Understanding the fundamentals of survey design can arm the researcher with the tools to design a good survey full of useful information.

Concept Reinforcement

1. Of the listed mistakes made in survey question design, which one(s) have you experienced?

2. Of the three types of questions, open-ended, multiple choice, and yes-no, which type would take the most time in preparing a dataset for analysis? Explain.

3. In what situation would an open-ended question be better than a multiple choice question?

Chapter 21 - Answer Choices and Layout in Survey Construction

Chapter Objectives

- Describe the issue with categorical options
- Describe the concept of mutually exclusive

The construction of a survey is a critical part of the survey process. In order to build a good survey, the researchers must have clearly defined the goals of the survey and the types of data he wants to collect from the subjects. Since a survey consists of questions, the researchers must think carefully about each question. The survey respondents will all be asked the same questions, but may interpret them differently. For example, if you are asked the question: "Do you have a child in school?," you will interpret the question differently depending on whether you have children and the ages of your children. If you do not have children, you might answer "no," meaning that you do not have any children. If you have children who are too young or too old to be in school, you might answer "no." The response is the same, but the meaning is very different.

Categorical Options

One method researchers use to present clear questions to survey respondents is providing categorical options. The categories allow the researchers to limit the number of answer options, while still providing more than two choices to the respondent.

Categories may include ranges of values, such as income ranges or age ranges. Categories may also include groupings of specific items, descriptions, levels of agreement or disagreement, etc. The categories are established based upon the goals of the research. Some common categories used in epidemiology surveys include: age, occupation, education level, gender, income, race, and ethnicity. Time is also often used as a categorical option. Epidemiologic surveys will often ask about diseases, exposures or behaviors from the past.

Common Categorical Options	Example Category 1	Example Category 2
Time	1-5 years 6-10 years 11-15 years	< 30 days 30-45 days >45 days
Age	Infant Child Teenager Adult	0-5 years old 6-10 years old 11-15 years old 16 years and older
Education level	High School Some College College Graduate Graduate School	12 years 14 years 16 years 18 years 20 years or more.

Mutually Exclusive

Most survey questions ask respondents to give specific answers. If these answers do not overlap, they are called mutually exclusive. When developing questions for an epidemiology survey, it is important that the responses to questions are mutually exclusive. For example, a yes/no question will get a yes or no answer. If the answer is yes, the answer cannot also be no. This is called mutually exclusive. Another area where it is very important to ensure that answer options are mutually exclusive is when asking respondents to select a range of values that best represents their specific situation. This could be income, age, weekly exercise, or any other variable. If the values in the answer options overlap, respondents will not answer consistently: some will choose one option and others will choose the second option. This will make it difficult to make any conclusions about the study results because the data were not collected in a consistent manner. Notice the sample in the image below. The first question is not mutually exclusive. Values are repeated in more than one category. For example, the value $15,000 appears as an option in both answer "a" and answer "b." The second version of the question solves this problem by providing mutually exclusive answer categories.

Mutually Exclusive

Question with non-mutually exclusive answers
What option best describes the annual income of your household?

A. $0-$15,000
B. $15,000 - $30,000
C. $30,000 - $45,000
D. $45,000 - $60,000
E. Above $60,000

Question with mutually exclusive answers
What option best describes the annual income of your household?

A. $0-$15,000
B. $15,001 - $30,000
C. $30,001 - $45,000
D. $45,001 - $60,000
E. Above $60,000

Summary

One of the most important parts of designing and implementing a survey to collect epidemiologic data is ensuring that the questions asked will elicit the correct response from the respondent. The questions must be clearly stated. If the questions provide answer options, the categories must be clearly described and mutually exclusive. If the question is unclear, respondents will interpret it differently, resulting in inconsistent answers that compromise the quality of the data being collected. If the answer categories overlap, respondents may provide the "same" answer by using different categories, both of which are correct.

Concept Reinforcement

1. Explain why researchers use categorical options when collecting data from respondents.

2. Discuss a potential problem with using categorical options in surveys.

3. Explain mutually exclusive and discuss why it is important in question and survey development.

Chapter 22 - Survey Layout

Chapter Objectives

- List the key characteristics of layout
- Describe the use of space and length

For questionnaires that the participants fill out themselves, they need to be constructed for ease of understanding. Several things need to be thought about in the design stage. These include formatting options, question order, and appearance of individual pages.

Design of the Questionnaire

Two objectives should be accomplished through the design of the questionnaire. One is to increase the number of responses. The second objective is to reduce the number of questions skipped or answered incorrectly.

One misconception is that a paper-and-pencil questionnaire allows the participant to carefully read the questions and answer them at their own speed. However, people really do not read the entire questionnaire in a thoughtful way. They use clues from the layout about what can be read and what can be ignored. It is not uncommon for participants to skip words. The best strategy is to keep the wording and visuals simple.

Grouping of Questions

A flow of questions in a survey is similar to the flow of a conversation. One rule of thumb is to group questions by topic. For example, put all the physical activity questions together.

One of the most important ways to get people to answer a survey is to have them feel it is relevant to them. In other words, if they feel the survey is asking about something that is important to them or interesting to answer, they are more likely to fill it out. It is impossible to have the entire questionnaire filled with terribly interesting questions—-some will be interesting to the participant and others less so. Therefore, the order to the question must also be carefully taken into consideration.

Rules of Thumb for Ordering of Questions

In the cover letter that accompanies a survey, the purpose of the questionnaire is described. Consequently, the first questions should directly speak to this purpose. For example, if the survey is about physical activity, the first questions should be about physical activity. Later questions can be about other important items such as age, sex, education attainment, and income level. Questions that ask about opinions or attitudinal scales should go in the middle of the survey. Concrete questions that just report facts, such as age and income should go at the end of the survey.

Besides these rules of thumb for placement of questions, questions should be order in a manner that seems logical to the participant. Generally, it helps to ask first details about an event before asking the participant to evaluate the event. For example, it makes sense to first ask about a medical condition, say a broken leg. First, ask about when, how and type of break. It would make sense to follow this with questions evaluating the medical care received.

Sources of Order Effects

We have lots of information on how the order of the questions can influence answers. There are 5 issues that a researcher should be aware of when designing a questionnaire. Depending on the ordering of the questions, big differences in responses can be seen.

Evenhandedness

This is a value-based response. People usually want to be fair. A survey done in 1948 tested question order. Some participants were asked first whether it is OK for an American reporter to write about a visit to the Soviet Union (now known as the USSR, Union of Soviet Socialist Republics). Some participants were asked whether it is OK for a communist reporter to write about a visit to the United States. When the first question was the communist reporter question, the percent of positive responses to the American reporter question was 37%. In contrast, when the first question was the American reporter question, the positive response to the American reporter was 73%. The order changed the responses by almost fifty percent. This is an example of even-handedness. Participants want to be even-handed in their responses so when put in a position of noticing this, for example how they treated a communist and American reporter, they may alter their answers.

Anchoring

This is a cognitive-based question. The first question influences the answer to the second question. In 1993, a survey was given to students with two questions about cheating in university. One question was asked about cheating in their university and the other asked about cheating in universities throughout the U.S. The order to the question changed the responses. If students were asked about cheating in U.S. universities first, they were much more likely to say that cheating was a problem at their university. This shows that the answer to the first question served as a reference point or anchor to the second question.

McCarthyism

During the late 1940s through the 1950s many thousands of Americans were accused of being Communists or communist sympathizers. Investigations into people's lives were conducted. The people singled out were often government employees, entertainers, teachers and union activist. The proof of communism or communist sympathy was often weak or almost non-existent. Many people lost their jobs, had their careers destroyed, especially those in the entertainment business, and sometimes wnet to prison. Almost all of the prison sentences were overturned later. However, the loss of a career could not be fixed later.

Carryover, subtraction, and summary item effect

The order of general questions followed immediately before or after a specific question influences the response. These can go in either direction and depend on the type of question. Sometimes, people maintain the same feeling from one question to another (e.g., question about one's marriage and then marriage in general). Sometimes, survey responders consider their response(s) to previous questions to adjust the answer to the more general question.

The First Question

No other question is more important than the first question since this one question can play a role in whether the respondent completes the questionnaire or throws it away. There are a few rules of thumb regarding this question. First, the question should apply to everyone who gets the survey. It should be linked to the purpose of the survey, as stated in the invitation letter and be interesting. It should be an easy question. For example, listing all people in your household is a lot harder than indicating the number of people in your household.

Page Design

According to Dillman, a leading researcher on survey design, many things can be done to improve a survey. Below are several pointers.

- Increasing font size helps attract attention
- Bolding helps attract attention
- Use spacing to group items
- Use similar font type to group items
- Begin asking questions in the upper right quadrant of the page
- Avoid use of the lower left quadrant
- Number the questions consistently
- Place more space between questions than between the question and answer options
- Use darker font for the question and lighter font for answer choices
- Vertical placement of answer choices is preferred
- If use horizontal placement of answer choices, all choices should be evenly spaced on one line

Cover Pages

The front cover page will be seen first. A well-designed cover can motivate someone to answer the questions. Simple graphics are better than detailed ones since a detailed one may contain errors or be annoying to the respondents. The title and name and address of investigator are included for easy reference.

The back cover is often white space. This is a place to invite comments, give a thank you. The back cover should not compete with the front cover.

Summary

Many pieces need to be considered for a survey to look professional. Additionally, the design can also influence participants' response. A poorly designed survey is more likely to be put aside and not completed compared to a well designed survey. Besides the design, understanding how people fill out surveys can help researchers design a survey to maximize participation.

Concept Reinforcement

1. In a survey asking about risk factors associated with quitting high school, what should be the first question?

2. Of all the things to think about in survey design, what do you think is the most important? Explain.

3. What is a possible example of a question in whichh even-handedness might play a role?

Chapter 23 - Use of Incentives and Participation Proportion

Chapter Objectives

- Describe the types of incentives

- List the pros and cons of using incentives

- Define participation proportion

- Explain the importance of participation proportion

Participation Proportion

All epidemiology studies published in peer reviewed journals spend some time informing the reader of the selection criteria for participation. Included in this description is the participation proportion (it is also commonly known as response rate; as a side note this term is technically incorrect since the term rate is a special kind of proportion often associated with frequency.)

Participation proportion is typically reported as a percent. It is the percent of people who agree to be in the study. Generally, a participation proportion over 70% is considered good in epidemiology studies. Twenty years ago, participation proportion of 90% was not uncommon. However, these days, less people are willing to participate in studies, it seems.

It is always important to figure out if the people who agree to be in the study are different in some important way from those who refuse to be in a study. Even if the sampling method is random, the results may not be generalizable if the characteristics of those who participate differ from those who do not participate. Some general characteristics of the non-responders may be known, and therefore compared with participants such as age and sex. The more characteristics that can be compared the better. For example, if a researcher is interested in describing quit attempts by smokers and no heavy smokers participated in the study, than even with a very good research plan, the results could not be generalized to all smokers since one subgroup—the long-term heavy smokers—did not provided data. Unless the researcher was able go gather this information, somehow, a mistake might be made in reporting the study results by thinking the results apply to all kinds of smokers.

Incentives

There are many studies that have looked at the ways to improve participation proportion in mailed surveys. Some of the findings make sense whereas others are less intuitive.

Money

One of the most powerful ways to improve participation proportion is to give respondents cash. It is not known how much cash makes a difference. Having $1 included in the mailed survey may be just as good as having $5. However, $20 would definitely increase the number of people who responded.

Besides just giving money, it is better to give people money as opposed to giving people money, if they fill out the survey. This is known as conditional incentive. In other words, the respondents will get the money, if they do something first.

Delivery

How the survey is delivered makes a difference. Special delivery can increase participation proportion 2-fold. Including a stamped return envelop as opposed to a preprinted business reply envelop increases response.

Using a window envelop or a larger envelop makes no difference. Similarly sending the survey to the work address versus the home address does not seem to make a difference. Using commemorative stamps also does not seem to change the percent of people who respond to the survey.

Sender

If the sender is from a university compared to the government or business, the participation increases. Surveys from physicians versus a research group shows no difference. The ethnicity of the sender has no influence on participation proportion. If the introductory letter is signed by senior or more well know person does not change the number of respondents. However, the introductory letter signed by hand versus computer generated signature seems to slightly increase the participation proportion.

Reminders

Sending a postcard or letter to let people know a survey is coming, called prenotification, improves participation proportion. The means of prenotification do not matter—either by telephone or by mail have the same participation proportion. Sending a second questionnaire helps improve participation proportion. Mentioning in the introductory letter that the respondents will be contacted again, if they do not fill out the questionnaire has no influence.

Content

It makes sense that a survey that is more interesting to the respondent is likely to be completed. Naturally, shorter questionnaires are more likely to be filled out than longer questionnaires. Questionnaires starting with relevant questions, easier, and more general questions at the beginning are more likely to be filled out.

Surveys with open ended questions where the respondent has to write the answer is less likely to be completed compared to closed questions (e.g., choosing from option list). Of course asking sensitive questions are less likely to be filled out. It does not matter whether the answer options are listed in increasing order or whether there are circles or check boxes.

Summary

Researchers strive to have high participation proportion so that they can state their findings with confidence. Physicians are well known for being very reluctant to fill out surveys. It is common to have 20% participation proportion for a physician survey. In cases where the participation proportion is low, the researcher always worries about how closely the respondents look like the non-respondents. Are the respondents different in some important way? Some research has gone into figuring out ways to maximize participation. Playing attention to all aspects of the data collection can make a different.

Concept Reinforcement

1. Why do you think people are less willing to participate in studies these days?

2. What would you consider sensitive question that your peer group would be reluctant to answer? How about your parents peer group?

3. Are there any sensitive questions that transcend generations?

4. What are the trade-offs between filling out the survey and not responding?

Chapter 24 - Biomarker Matrices and Collection

Chapter Objectives

- Explain matrices and general collection protocols
- List five advantages of using biomarkers
- List disadvantages of using biomarkers

Epidemiology uses mathematical formulas to show the relation between exposure and dis-ease outcome. In this chapter we are going to explore the use of **biomarkers,** which are measures of exposure in biological samples used to quantify exposure.

Exposure

In the early examples of epidemiology, researchers did not know exactly what **factors** or **agents** were associated with a disease. For example, Dr. Snow did not know what caused people to get sick with cholera. He used epidemiology tools, such as maps and interviews, to help him compile evidence that the agent was something in the water. He actually died before learning about the discovery of the bacillus that caused cholera. The cholera bacillus was discovered in 1854 by an Italian anatomist, Fillip Pacini. Unfortunately, Pacini did not prove that the bacillus that he discovered caused the disease, so his work remained obscure, and his reports were not translated into English.

In epidemiology, most of the early cases showing a relation between exposure and health status occurred in occupational settings. Often the exposure to the agent is much higher in occupational settings compared to the general population. In addition, the agent is also more readily identified in the occupational setting than in the general population.

Below are some examples of diseases associated with exposure. Both magnitude of exposure to the agent and identity of the agent are more readily obvious in occupational settings.

- Black lung disease associated with coal mining (inhaling coal dust).
- Mad hatters disease (insanity) associated with working in the millinery (hat) trade where mercury nitrate was used to treat the felt lining of hats.
- Chimney sweeps and testicular cancer (coal tar).
- Clock dial painters and bone cancer (paint was laced with radium 226 so that the dials glowed).

Even though the association of exposure to disease was eventually clear to the general public, the cause of the disease often remained unknown for some time.

Exposure has four components.

- A target, such as a person.

- An agent, such as plasmodium (parasite that causes malaria).

- The vector: The means of getting the agent to the target. A classic example of a vector is the mosquito. In some cases, in place of the vector is the environment. For example, air is the "vector" for transmitting ozone.

- Contact between the target and the agent. In the malaria case, the contact is a bite from the infected mosquito.

Exposure has also been strongly associated with **dose**. A common phrase in **toxicology**, or some would say a basic rule, is "the dose makes the poison."

A 16th century Swiss chemist, Paracelsus, is credited with this rule. The concept is that practically every substance on earth (including water and vitamin C) can kill a person if it is concentrated enough in a person's stomach or blood stream.

Biomarkers

Biomarkers are cellular, biochemical, or molecular alterations that are measurable in biological media, e.g., human tissue, cells, or fluids.

Three types of measurement are used for biomarkers:

- The level of the substance itself in biological media

- The level of products of **bio-transformation** of the substances in the same media. For example DDT is the substance that people are exposed to but once in the body it is transformed into DDE.

- The biological effect that result from contact of the external agent with the human body

Advantages to Using Biomarkers in Epidemiology Studies

1. Improve study validity and reduce bias in data

This means that the researcher is much more confident that the exposure really happened. Remember back to Chapter 4 on self reported data and recall bias. Determining the level of the agent in the biological sample is much stronger evidence of exposure than when someone reports that s/he was exposed

2. More nuanced measurements of the exposure

In today's scientific world, the level of detection is very low for many agents, in the parts per million, or parts per billion.

In general, the health effects of any toxic substance are related to the amount of exposure, also known as the dose. Generally, the greater the dose the person is exposed to, the more severe the effects from that exposure. Some chemicals can cause toxicity at very low doses and so it is important to be able to understand how these very small amounts are measured.

Concept Extension – Dose Measurement Systems

Parts per million (ppm) and parts per billion (ppb) are the most commonly used terms to describe very small amounts of contaminants (or agents) in **biospecimens**. They are measures of concentration, the amount of one material in a larger amount of another material. They are expressed as concentrations rather than total amounts. For example, researchers do not have to measure the total amount of lead in a person's entire blood supply to understand the level of exposure. They merely measure the concentration in a small sample to represent the total amount. In doing so, they can compare the concentration levels among the participants.

Sometimes, instead of using the part per million or billion terminology, concentrations are reported in weight units; such as the weight of the contaminant compared to the weight of the total. The metric system is often used. For example, a milligram is a thousandth of a gram and a gram is a thousandth of a kilogram. Therefore, a milligram is a thousandth of a thousandth, or a millionth of a kilogram. A milligram is one part per million of a kilogram. One part per million (ppm) is the same as one milligram per kilogram, mg/kg. In summary, one ppm equals one mg/kg.

In the metric weight system, a microgram is a thousandth of a milligram. Since a milligram is a millionth of a kilogram, and the microgram is a thousand times smaller, it is equivalent to a billionth of a kilogram. Microgram is abbreviated ug. Therefore, a part per billion is equal to a microgram per kilogram, ug/kg.

In the metric liquid measurement system, the unit of liquid volume most commonly used is the liter. A liter of water weighs one kilogram. If the contaminant is a solid, it is measured in milligrams. Thus, one part per million of a solid in a liquid can be written as a milligram per liter and abbreviated mg/l. Similarly, a part per billion of a solid in a liquid is equal to a ug/l.

Example: PCB Illustration of Dose Measurement

Polychlorinated biphenyls (PCBs) have been implicated in developmental deficiencies and neurologic problems in children, disruption of reproductive functions, liver disease, effects on the thyroid and immune system, and increased cancer risks. PCBs are synthetic organic compounds comprising 209 individual chlorinated biphenyl compounds (also known as **congeners**). Although the manufacture of PCBs was banned in the United States in the 1970s, people are still exposed to them. They are persistent compounds that degrade very slowly. It is important to understand the primary source of exposure. Below is a case study of PCB exposure from diet versus water.

In determining the important source of exposure, we will compare the relative importance of PCBs in Great Lakes fish consumption versus PCBs in Great Lakes drinking water consumption. The maximum level of PCBs legally allowed in fish sold in interstate commerce is 2 parts per million (ppm). (This does not apply to fish sold locally, however.) In contrast, the average PCB level of the Great Lakes drinking water is 4 parts per trillion (ppt). (No legal limit exists for drinking water level.)

Remember that a part per million is a million times more than a part per trillion. The fish levels are measured in ppm whereas the water levels are measured in ppt. So at first, one would assume that the fish consumption is a more important source of PCBs than the water consumption. However, it is not only the concentration level but also the dose—how much is consumed that is also important.

We consume a lot more water than fish on a daily basis. For example, a few people might eat as much as a pound of fish a day or as little as one pound every 6 months (180 days). On the other hand, people generally drink at least 2-4 liters (4-8 pounds) of water a day.

For those who drink little (4 lb/day) and eat lots of fish (1lb/day), it is clear that fish is the largest source of PCBs. Exposure from great lakes water consumption is 4 parts per trillion versus the exposure from eating fish, which is 1 part per billion. The same holds true for heavy water drinkers (8 pounds/day) and light fish eaters (1/180 lb per day). For this group, the PCB exposure from great lakes water is 8 parts per trillion and from fish it is 0.006 (1 ÷ 180) parts per billion. So fish consumption, even for people who rarely eat fish is most likely the main source of exposure. Consequently, if a PCB advisory was posted, the advisory would target fish consumption and not drinking water consumption.

3. Identify individual susceptibility, e.g., genetic biomarkers

Example: PKU Illustration

In 1934, a Norwegian doctor, Asbjorn Folling, discovered the cause of severe mental retardation in 2 young children, PKU (phenylketonuria), also known as Folling's Disease in Norway after the discoverer. PKU is called an error of metabolism because children cannot break down phenylalanine, an **amino acid** making up approximately 5% of all protein foods. Dr. Folling showed that PKU was an inherited disease. At that time, the prevalence of PKU in institutions for severely mentally retarded individuals in western counties was 1-2%. Blood tests were developed in the early 1960s to test for this genetic abnormality since, if caught early–within the first 2 weeks of life–mental retardation can often be prevented. In the United States, the newborn screening test for PKU is mandated by law in all states except Maryland and Wyoming.

Example: BCRA 1 and 2

A history of breast cancer in **first-degree relatives** is an important breast cancer risk factor, particularly if the cancer occurred at an early age. Some breast cancers that cluster in families are associated with inherited mutations in particular genes, such as BRCA1 or BRCA2. BRCA stands for BReast CAncer one and two.

BRCA1 and BRCA2 are major genes related to hereditary breast cancer; they were discovered in 1994 and 1995 respectively. BRCA1/2-affected women carry a high risk of developing breast cancer, ovarian cancer, melanoma, and pancreatic cancer. BRCA1/2-affected men have an increased risk of also developing breast cancer, pancreatic cancer, melanoma, and prostate cancer.

Commercial genetic testing to identify people who have the mutations in the BRCA1 and BRCA2 genes is now readily available. However, unlike PKU, there is no treatment for BRCA1 and BRCA2 to decrease the cancer risks.

4. Allows for early detection of disease or illness

Example: HDL cholesterol and atherosclerosis.

Atherosclerosis is known as hardening of the arteries. Complications of atherosclerosis are the leading cause of death in the United States. Atherosclerosis can be considered to be a form of chronic inflammation. Michael S. Brown and Joseph L. Goldstein received the Nobel Prize in Physiology or Medicine in 1985 for their discoveries about the regulation of cholesterol metabolism and treatment of diseases caused by elevated levels of cholesterol in the blood.

Commercial cholesterol testing is available to identify people with **HDL**, "good" cholesterol and **LDL**, "bad" cholesterol. Statins are the current drug of choice to lower the LDL levels.

5. Provides a clue as to the mechanism of disease occurrence

Example: Hepatitis C

Hepatitis C is the leading cause of liver transplants. It is a blood-borne infectious viral disease. It is usually spread through contact with infected blood. Most people with hepatitis C do not have any symptoms. There is no cure for hepatitis C.

Biomarkers are used to predict a hepatitis C liver transplant patient's chance of developing fibrosis, a formation of scar-like tissue that can lead to cirrhosis. Changes in certain types of liver cells are useful in determining those who are at the greatest risk for developing fibrosis.

6. Provides data on effectiveness of intervention trials

Example: Isocyanate Exposure

Automobile painters can be exposed to hardeners that are part of the topcoat of automobile paints. These hardeners contain isocyanate resins. Workers exposed to isocyanate may develop a serious or fatal respiratory disease. An intervention to decrease isocyanate exposure to workers in automobile body shops used urinary biological monitoring (urine testing) of exposure. Workers provided a urine specimen after work each day. In shops that had ventilation fans turned on all the time, workers were found to have lower isocyanate level.

Disadvantages of Biomarkers

1. There can be considerable variation in levels biomarkers within a person depending on time of day or month.

Example: melatonin

Melatonin, a neurohormone, is produced from the amino acid tryptophan, in the brain by the pineal gland. Melatonin's synthesis and release increases in the absence of light, i.e., at night or in darkness. Based on this characterization, melatonin is involved in circadian rhythm and regulations of diverse body functions.

2. There can be considerable variation in the levels of biomarkers between people that is not related to the disease outcome.

Example: menstrual blood loss for moderate or less severe periods and anemia

Menstrual length has significant variation among women with an average of 3-7 days and the amount of blood loss can be qualitatively described as light, moderately light, moderate, moderately heavy, and heavy. In studies, the intensity of a woman's period measured in blood loss was not associated with anemia for women in all categories, except heavy menstrual periods (>120mL).

3. Considerable intra-individual variation (variation from one sample to another in the same person).

Example: total mercury in blood

Developmental deficits in children associated with mercury exposure are well documented. Pregnant women and young children are advised to limit fish consumption due to this health effect. Total mercury in plasma is associated with both inorganic mercury and organic mercury with large inter-individual variations in the distribution between red blood cells and plasma. The inter-individual variation in the blood to hair ratio is also very large.

4. Many exposures have a short half-life.

Example: Atrazine, a common corn herbicide

Atrazine exposure can occur during corn planting season. Two common ways that atrazine exposure can happen is by inhalation of suspended particles (drift) or ingested from touching food with hands contaminated with the pesticide and then eating the food or hand (contaminated with the pesticide) to mouth behavior. Atrazine's half life in urine is 24 hours. In 48 hours, all of the atrazine from the previous 48 hours will have been eliminated.

5. Gathering tissues or fluids to analyze them for contaminants can be intrusive.

Fear of needles, known as belonephobia, is a condition in which an individual is extremely afraid of facing needles or injections. It has been reported that up to 10% of the population has a state of apprehension when facing the possibility of a needle stick. Consequently, gathering blood is considered significantly more intrusive than most other forms of biospecimen collections such as toenail collection, urine collection, or saliva collection.

6. Both gathering biospecimens and analyzing them for contaminants is costly.

Current instrumentation allows for detection of minute levels of biomarkers in specimens. However, with the more precise detection a cost is associated with these analyses.

Summary

Perhaps one of the most fundamental problems in epidemiology is measuring the exposure. For example, cell phone use has been linked to increased risk of brain cancer in some but not all epidemiology studies. Typically, the exposure is ascertained by asking study participants their usage of cell phones, duration and frequency. These indirect measures leave critical questions unanswered such as internal dose of the hazardous exposure. The use of biomarkers can, in some cases, provide reasonable data on exposure to the hazardous substance and thereby strengthen the study findings.

Concept Reinforcement

Explain how occupational exposure helps epidemiologists understand the effects of exposure to specific factor or agents in the population.

Discuss the advantages to using biomarkers to study population health. Discuss the disadvantages of using biomarkers in epidemiologic studies.

Chapter 25 - Making a Map – MAUP

Chapter Objectives

- Describe the modifiable area unit problem
- Describe the advantages of using map for data presentation
- Discuss the limitations of maps for representation of data

Everyone knows the adage, "A picture is worth a thousand words." The new adage is "a map is worth a thousand pictures." The imagery shown on a map is immediate and compelling. With the advent of user friendly desktop software to create maps and the electronic files provided by the US census bureau as well as other organizations, researchers can now display data using maps. When a map is created, it gives the impression of complete information. However, like any other type of presentation the quality of the information shown on a map is only as good as the completeness and accuracy of the data used to make the map.

One significant benefit of using a map is the ability of a map to portray complex information in an understandable way. Further, mapping can visually show the data table for ease of comprehension. Another benefit of maps are their universal appeal. A specific language is not needed but rather an understanding of universal symbols. Maps are also visually appealing and can be used to communicate results while also giving a reader a visual break from dense text. Maps can also reinforce information by visually showing results that are described in the text.

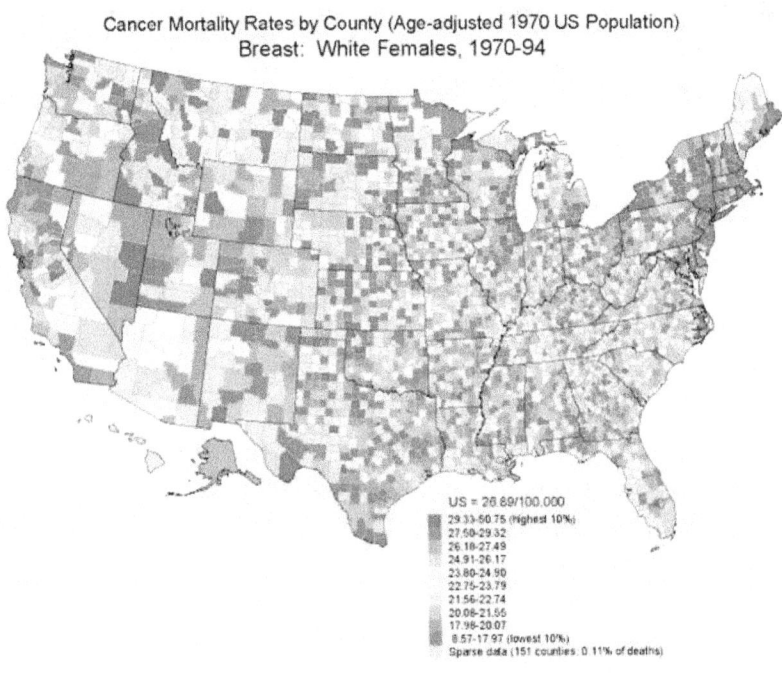

Geographic variation of breast cancer mortality by county;
http://www3.cancer.gov/atlasplus/

Map Limitations

There are several limitations to displaying data via maps. Areal bias is one limitation that can occur. The visual impact of a map is related to both shading and surface area. Surface area is the area represented by the areal unit, for example some states are much larger than others in square miles, but may represent a smaller population compared to a state with a smaller area, but denser population. Most of the New England states are geographically small but densely populated as compared to the many of the Mid-western states.

Look at the map below that shows the mortality rate by state for brain and nervous system cancer in white males, 1970 to 1994, all ages.

Without thinking, which states draw your attention? Again, looking quickly at the map, list the states with the highest mortality rates.

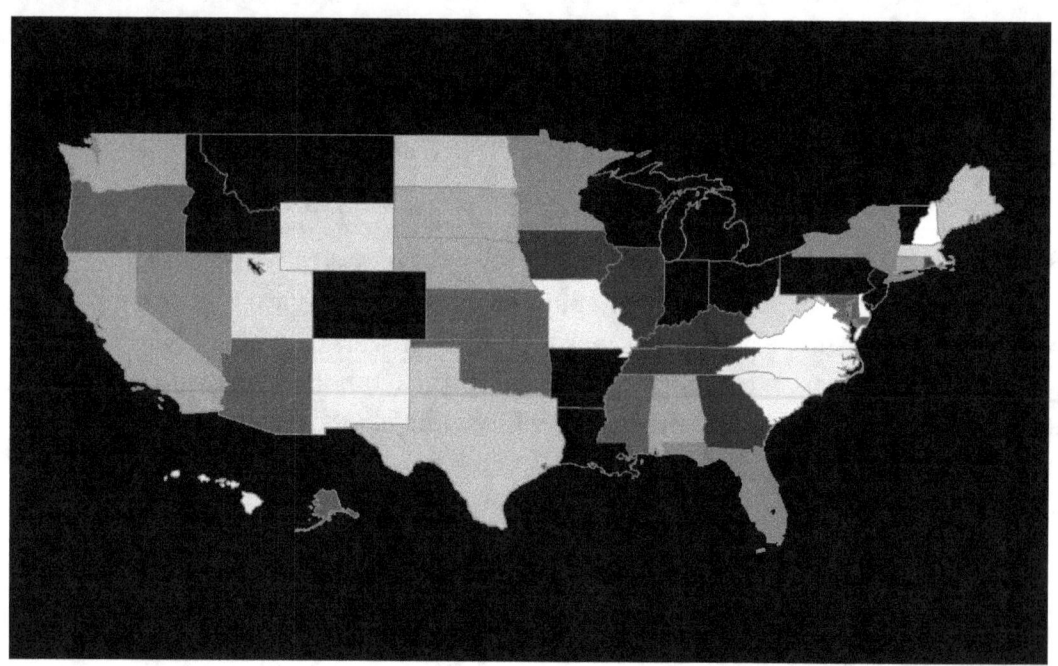

Brain and nervous system cancer mortality rates in white males, 1970 to 1994

> **Chloropleth**
> Maps that show information based on area (areal) units and use color to show data ranges.

If you are like most people, your eye will be drawn to the dark color. You will probably notice Idaho, Montana, and Colorado first as having high rates. These states are large in area and they are colored in black. This demonstrates the areal bias. New Jersey and New Hampshire also has very high brain cancer rates but these states are not noticed as quickly due to their geographic size.

A second limitation of maps is the **modifiable area unit problem** (MAUP). This means the results of a study can appear to change tremendously when showing these data on choropleth maps using different areal units.

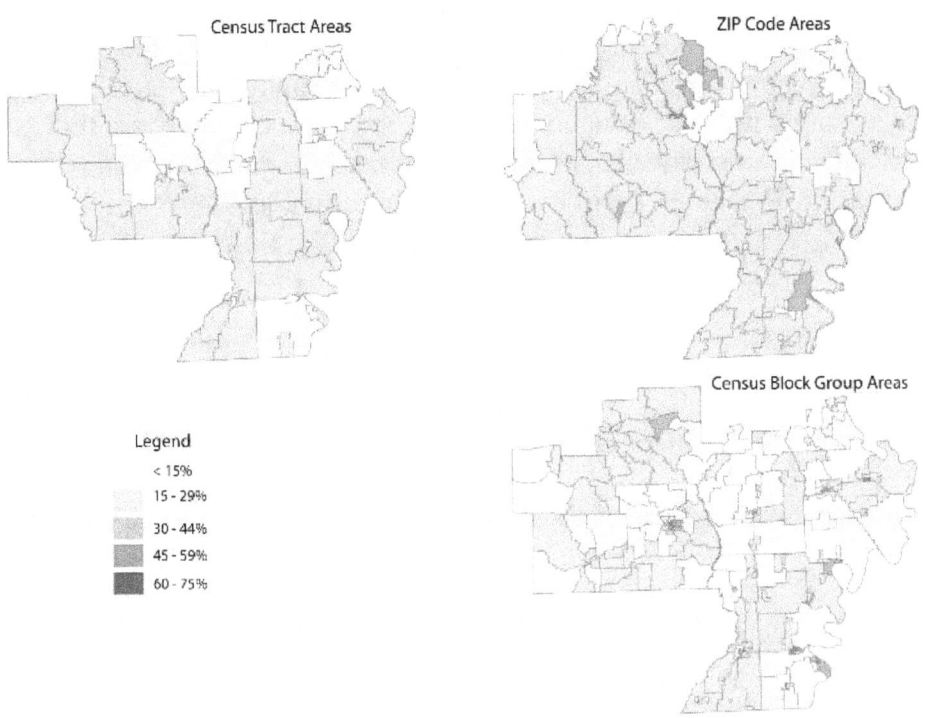

Percent of households with income < $10,000 shown by various areal units in the Bootheel region of Missouri

The third limitation of maps is the inability to show how confident the researcher is in the results. In tables, researchers have ways to present the data that tells the reader the confidence of the findings. However, there has not been any system developed to do the same thing with maps.

Summary

Although a map must by its very nature distort reality since the 3-dimensional world is portrayed on a 2-dimensional surface, the researcher needs to be attentive to the construction of the map. With the availability of user-friendly mapping software, cartography is no longer left to those with a background in this science. Although there are limitations in the use of maps, there are also advantages. Mapping is becoming more and more popular in the visual display of data with the goal of universal understanding.

Concept Reinforcement

1. Why do you think a map seems to be more believable than written results.

2. What educational experiences support the use of maps to convey knowledge.

3. For the most part, the data shown on a map is taken as being 100% true; however, this is rarely the case. In data analysis, there is always so degree of uncertainty. How would you portray uncertainty on a map?

Chapter 26 - Chloropleth Maps

Chapter Objectives

- Define the features of a chloropleth map
- Define the ways to categorize data
- Explain the assumptions made on color

Maps are powerful tools used to communicate information. There are many types of maps that an epidemiologist can use. One of the most common types of map is, choropleth maps. Choropleth maps are based on predefined areal units, such as states, counties, census tracts, etc. These areas are filled with color that symbolizes ranges in values from the data.

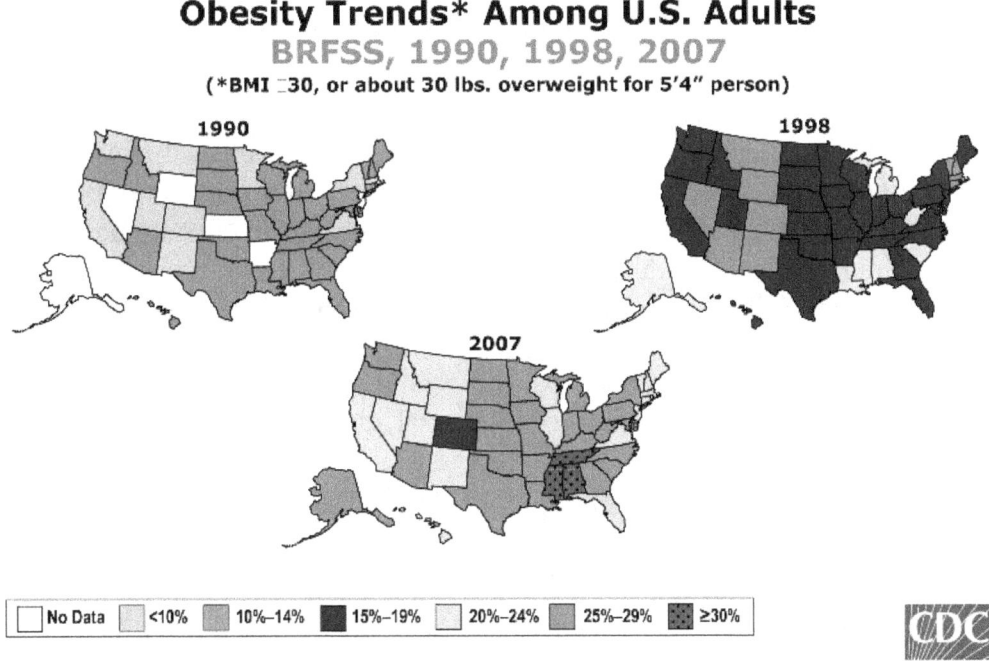

Obesity trends by state in 1990, 1998 and 2007

The obesity map is a choropleth map. It uses states as the areal unit. BMI means body mass index. It is the calculation that uses height and weight to classify people as underweight, normal, overweight and obese.

$$BMI = \frac{(\text{weight in pounds} \times 703)}{\text{height in inches}^2}$$

Body mass index calculation

Constructing a Choropleth Map

Three fundamental decisions need to be made when constructing a map. These are deciding about areal units, color selection and data classing. Data classing means how to organize the data into categories.

Areal Unit Selection

Depending on the data, the areal unit may be predetermined. For example, if the researcher has data on county level smoking rates, then these data can be displayed at the county level or shown at a regional or state level. The data will determine the scale used to map these data. Data can always be aggregated up but not the other way. For example, if the researcher has county level data, these data cannot be displayed at the town level because all the cities and towns in the county will have the same value.

Color Selection

For sequential values, the general rule of thumb is to order the color of the data from light to dark to parallel the ordering of the low to high values. The other type of data is bifurcated. This is also known as diverging data. It may have an obvious structure such as positive and negative numbers with zero as the middle value. It is common for high values to be shown in red and low values to be shown in blue. A less common color scheme in epidemiology is qualitative. Qualitative colors use a rainbow scheme that purposely has no pattern. The range of qualitative colors is useful for categories in which the data are descriptive. For example, qualitative colors could be used to show means of getting to school by neighborhoods in a city (e.g., walk/bike, automobile, public bus, commuter rail/train). Dr. Cynthia Brewer developed color schemes for sequential, diverging and qualitative categories

Dr. Brewer has provided color schemes for sequential, diverging and qualitative categories. These are available on her web site.

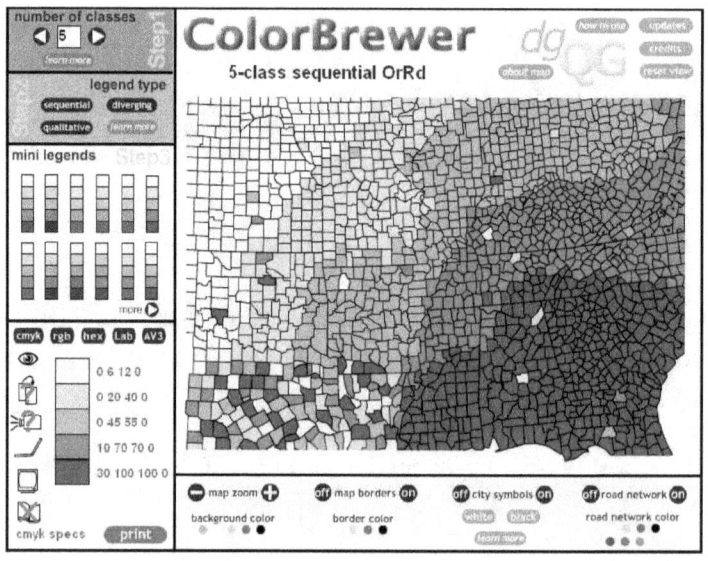

Color Brewer site, www.colorbrewer.org/

When choosing colors for use in maps, it is very important to consider the impact of the colors on the reader of the map. Some key considerations are whether certain intensities cause the reader to place higher or lower importance on the data represented by that color, as well as maintaining an awareness that color blind people's limitations.

In what media the map will be viewed must also be taken into consideration when choosing colors. If it is anticipated that the map will be copied using black and white print, some color scheme maintain their differentiation in values while others do not. Similarly, attention needs to be paid to color choice when the map is projected (LCD use), color printed, or displayed on a laptop.

Color preferences vary by culture and other characteristics. However, little is known about the effects of preference on map interpretation. Even without support from research studies, map designers can use color in an obvious or clever way to reinforce the map message. For example, adding a gold outline to a dollar sign can reinforce the idea of wealth.

Categories Selection

Another basic decision when constructing a map is how to break up the data into categories. Categorizing the data differently can tell very different stories. There is no right way to categorize the data. However, a perceptive reader will pay close attention to this detail when looking at the map.

Common ways to class data are as follows:

Quantiles: This is putting equal number of areal units into each class. For example, there are 72 counties in Wisconsin. If six categories are chosen, the quantiles will each have 12 counties.

Equal interval: This breaks up the data ranges into equal segments. In other words, the entire range of data values from minimum to maximum value is divided equally into however many categories have been chosen. In this situation, the number of counties could vary tremendously between classes since the data values determine in which category the county will be placed.

In a hypothetical map of percent land in mixed zoning, the quantile and equal interval breaks distribute the data quite differently. Mixed zoning is neighborhoods with two or more of the following types of land use: industry, commerce, residential, resource protected, and municipality.

	Quantiles		Equal Interval	
	Towns	Ranges	Towns	Ranges
Class 1	A-M	0-13	A-F	1-2
Class 2	N-U	14-28	G-M	3-10
Class 3	V	29-42	N-S	15-25
Class 4	W-Z	43-56	T-Z	25-56

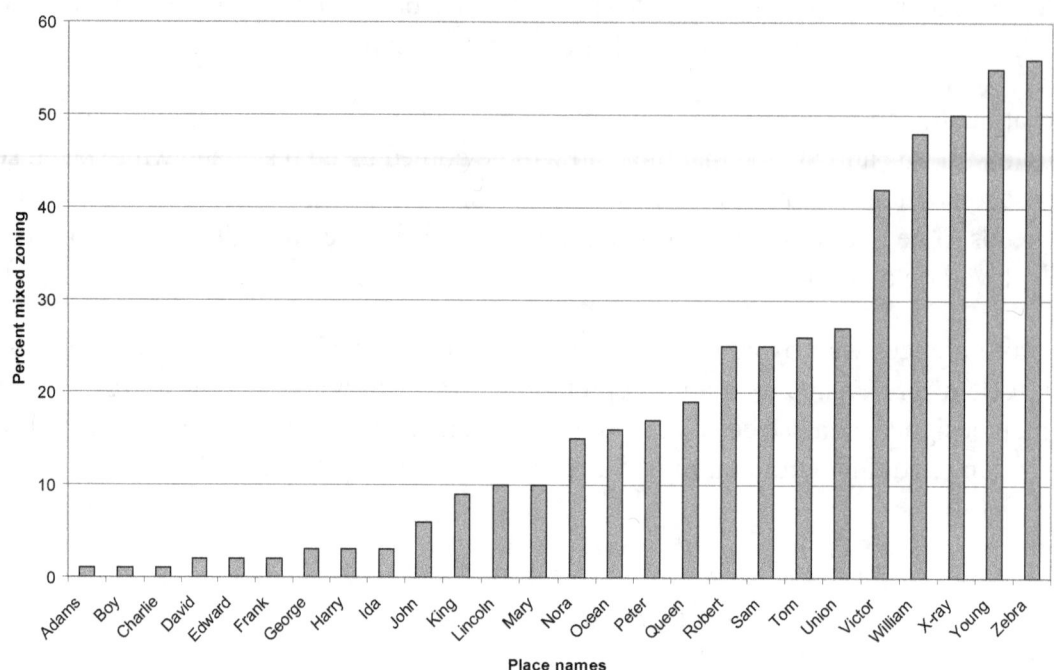

26 hypothetical towns showing percent of land with mixed zoning

Natural breaks (also known as Jenks breaks) minimize the variation *within* the classes and maximize the variation *between* classes. This system is close to the quantile system but adds some mathematical calculation to improve the fit.

Below are three maps of exactly the same data using the same color scheme: mortality rate by state for brain and nervous system cancer in white males, 1970 to 1994, all ages. Notice how the story changes for Idaho with the different classing system.

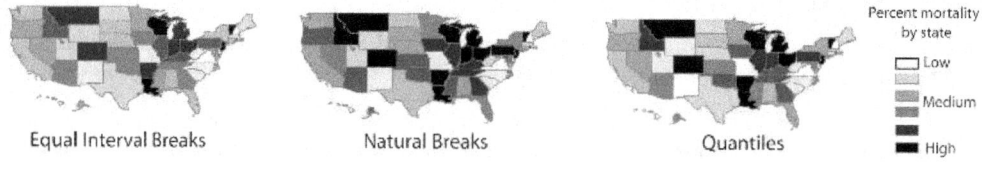

Mortality rate by state for brain and nervous system cancer in white males, 1970 to 1994, all ages

Summary

Chloropleth maps are a specific type of map used by epidemiologists to display ranges of values using color within specified areal units. Chloropleth maps contain standard map components, as well as definitions of the areal units and the color schemes used to represent the ranges of values. The ranges of values are classed using different schemes, each of which is likely to produce a different looking map. In general, color is used from light to dark based on lowest to highest values for the data. It is important to be careful, however, to make sure the intensity of the color will communicate well to the reader the importance of the parts of the map containing that color. It is also important to keep in mind the limitations some people have in seeing color, such as those who are color blind.

Concept Reinforcement

1. What does the color red mean to you? In other words, do you think it makes more sense to show high values or low values using the color red? How about blue?

2. Does it worry you at all to know that the way the categories are divided can actually change the look of a map? What could an epidemiologist do to present the data in the unbiased way?

3. What is it about mapping that makes it so appealing to use in displaying results?

Chapter 27 - Making a Map – Elements

Chapter Objectives

- List three features of a map

- Describe the difference in vector versus pixel data

Epidemiologists are not cartographers, people who specialize in map making. However, map making is becoming more and more common in the world of epidemiology. Of course, John Snow's cholera map is shown in practically every introductory epidemiology book.

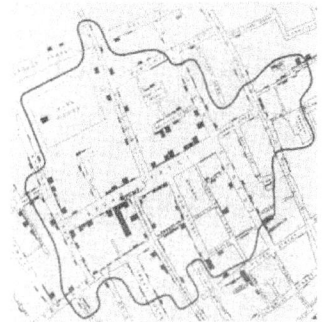

Soho area of London showing cholera deaths in 1854

Another series of maps that has received wide appeal are the obesity maps produced by Centers of Disease Control and Prevention (CDC).

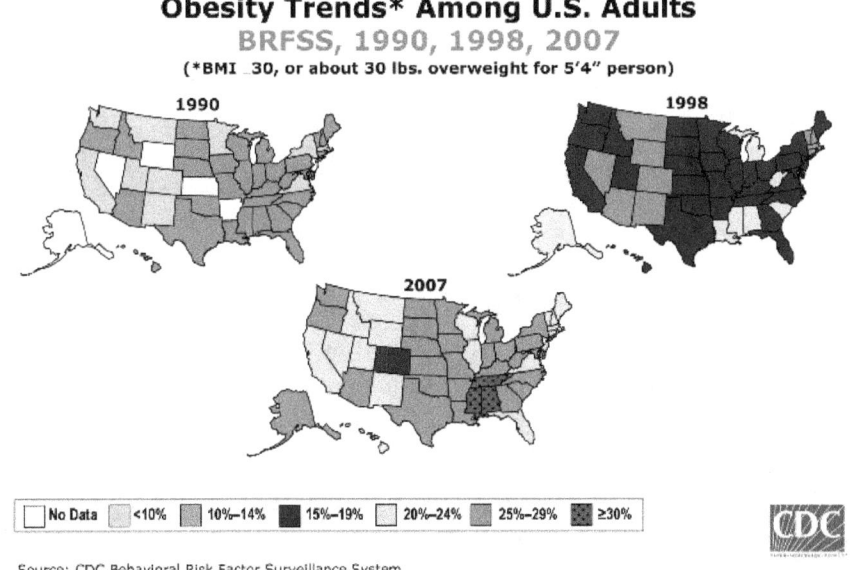

Obesity trends by state in 1990, 1998 and 2007

All maps are made of three components: points, lines and polygons. Mixing these components in sensible ways forms the bases of creating a well designed map. The purpose of a well designed map is to show the reader what is the most important piece of information. The epidemiologist thinks about the elements of the map to be noticed first and what elements to be remembered. Map makers think about this visual hierarchy or ordering of importance. Maps are designed so that some parts appear to be background material and some parts are prominent, in the foreground.

Components of a Map

The title is one of the most prominent elements in a map. It should stand alone in describing the map meaning. In other words, a person should be able to read the title and understand what the map is showing without having to read any additional descriptions in the text.

The legend tells the reader how the data are categorized. How the data are divided into categories is extremely important since the meaning can change depending on how the data are displayed.

In epidemiology, a direction arrow should be included if it is not obvious. North is assumed to be the top of the page and therefore if a map is oriented in the same direction, a direction arrow is optional. In contrast, cartographers feel that a direction arrow is integral to a map. Therefore, placement of the direction arrow is at the discretion of the map maker but probably should not be very prominent.

The scale bar is identical to the direction arrow. This tells the reader the linear distance, the scale. This is a typical component of a map when the image is not common, though in epidemiology this piece of information is often omitted since it is rare that distance is the point of the map. In contrast, cartographers considered this a necessary component of maps.

Once a map has been make with user friendly software, it is exported in an appropriate file format. Two general types of file formats are raster and vector.

Raster Versus Vector Images

Raster images are composed of a grid of pixels. Each pixel has a specific color value assigned to it. A pixel is usually very small so that a seemingly smooth image is created. If this raster image is magnified, then the individual boxes in the grid can be seen. Consequently, a raster image has an optimal viewing size.

A computer screen generally shows 72 pixels per inch and most printers work with 600-2400 pixels per inch. The term ppi, pixels/inch, dots/inch, samples/inch, or spi all mean the same thing.

In contrast, vector images use mathematical formulas to describe shapes. Because of this, there is no optimal size of a vector image. The image can be printed or displayed at the highest resolution of the device such as a computer screen or printer.

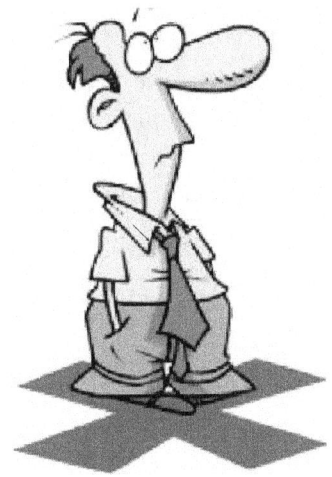

Clip art image of a man

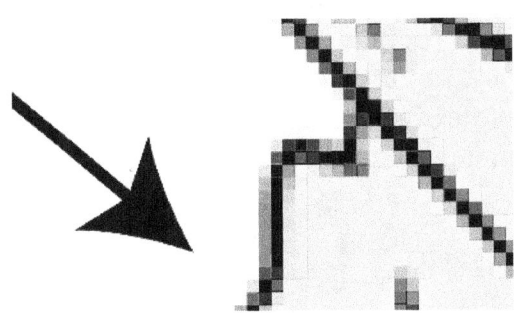

Blowup of clip art image of man: the arrow is vector and the man's shirt is raster

On a map, these two types of images are displayed differently depending on the map component of a point, line or polygon.

	Vector	Raster
Point	●	☐
Line	—	▭▭▭▭▭
Polygon	☐	▦

Comparison of the vector and raster data

Advantages of Raster and Vector Images

Advantages of vector images include the resolution of the image is independent of the size. The outline of an image is also smooth. Compared to raster images, the file size is smaller.

Advantages of raster images is that this in the only format that will show subtle gradients of color and details. Raster images also allow color correction much easier than a vector image.

Summary

In a presentation of study results, a map may only be one part of the presentation. In contrast, the map may tell the whole story. For example, the series of maps about obesity that the Centers for Disease Control and Prevention (CDC) provide compelling evidence about the United States obesity epidemic. One of the most important lessons a beginning mapmaker learns is to know the purpose of the map. In other words, what the map is supposed to tell the viewer. Once that has been identified, the smart epidemiologist uses the different elements in a thoughtful way, confers with a cartographer, and uses resource books written to help non-map making profession create a map. Even a design professional can assist in the choice of colors to communicate the purpose of the map.

Concept Reinforcement

1. What choices were made in the obesity maps with regard to basic components of a map?

2. Do you think the obesity maps would be as compelling if counties were used as the areal unit instead of states? (There are on average 62 counties per state with Delaware only having 3 and Texas having 254.)

3. Do you think a direction arrow or a scale should have been included on the obesity map? Explain

Chapter 28 - Use of Tables in Reporting Results

Chapter Objectives

- State five standard features of a table.
- Describe the purpose of a table.
- Describe the elements necessary for clear table heading and title

Epidemiologists collect data, analyze it, and present it. From all that work, knowledge may come. Tables are used to present data. A well-constructed table communicates to the reader the essence of the study. In medium to large studies, the first table in an article is a characteristics table. Information about the participants are summarized so that readers can find a description of the participants at a glance. Additional tables typically present study results or other details that are best shown in a tabular form.

Purpose of a Table

The general purpose of a table is to include important data beyond what can be simply reported in the text. The maximum size of a table should be no more than a single page, held as when reading the text. Because the maximum number of lines is significantly greater than the maximum number of columns, the data are displayed such that the greatest number of items is naturally assigned to the columns. The order of data in the table has considerable flexibility. Ordering is typically alphabetical, chronological, geographical or according to magnitude of the items. The most conspicuous position in a table is top and left.

> **Unambiguous**
> Clear. In terms of data, this means there is a clear result.

Rules of Thumb for Displaying Data

A table should tell us what the numbers represent and how the numbers were obtained or calculated. In other words, the table should be an efficient display of meaningful and unambiguous data.

The following table is adapted from a paper written by Jane McElroy and colleagues, called "Potential Exposure to PCBs, DDT, and PBDEs from Sport-Caught Fish Consumption in Relation to Breast Cancer Risk in Wisconsin. This paper was published in the journal, Environmental Health Perspectives in 2004.

Table 1. Characteristics of Women with Breast Cancer and Controls Aged 20-69 years

Characteristic	Cases (N=1456)		Controls (N=1276)	
	N	%	N	%
Age at reference date (years)				
< 40	104	7.1%	102	8.0%
40-49	389	26.7%	343	26.9%
50-54	263	18.1%	196	15.4%
55-59	255	17.5%	210	16.5%
60-64	240	16.5%	204	16.0%
65-69	205	14.1%	221	17.3%
Family history				
None	1142	78.4%	1100	86.2%
Positive‡	304	20.9%	168	13.2%
Unknown	10	0.7%	8	0.6%
Recent alcohol consumption				
None	243	16.7%	219	17.2%
1-6 drinks/week	1022	70.2%	931	73.0%
7 or more drinks/week‡	189	13.0%	126	9.9%
Parity				
0-1	342	23.5%	276	21.7%
2	467	32.1%	373	29.2%
3 or more‡	646	44.4%	626	49.1%
Age at First Birth (years old)				
< 20	236	16.2%	243	19.0%
20-24	613	42.1%	581	45.5%
25-29‡	297	20.4%	207	16.2%
≥30‡	131	9.0%	95	7.5%
Nulliparous	179	12.3%	150	11.8%
Age at menopause (years old)†				
<45	192	23.2%	205	27.6%
45-49	187	22.6%	170	22.9%
50-54	233	28.2%	219	29.5%
55-69‡	95	11.5%	65	8.8%
Unknown	119	14.3%	84	11.3%
Education				
< High School diploma	75	5.2%	83	6.5%
High School diploma	621	42.7%	534	41.9%
Some College	388	26.7%	356	27.9%
College degree	366	25.1%	300	23.5%
Unknown	6	0.4%	3	0.2%

* Adjusted for age.
† Among postmenopausal women only.
‡ Statistically significant

Researchers generally display data in a similar fashion. There are several rules of thumb for displaying data in a table.

In constructing a table, the names of the columns and rows should be clear and short. In addition, subordinate information should be indented. In the example table above, all the characteristics are listed at the far left edge of the table. The categories of the characteristics are all indented to spaces.

One of the first overarching rules of thumb is that the table should be understandable by itself. In other words, it can stand alone. In the example above, the title tells the reader that information in this table is comparing two groups of women—women with and without breast cancer. Several demographics about these women are compared by stating the number and percent of women in each category.

Another rule of thumb is the data in a table are closely related to other data in the table. The reader can look at the table and summarize the facts. In the example above, all the data are about differences and similarities in lifestyle choices and risk factors associated with breast cancer.

Next, column and row headings should be brief, unambiguous, and self-explanatory. Table footnotes should be used only to enhance the clarity of the headings. The symbol † means among postmenopausal women only. This makes sense for the characteristic describing age at menopause. Although the row heading should be clear, in this case, "age of menopause" meaning that it could only apply to women who have gone through menopause, the symbol linked to the footnote adds clarity.

Any variation in the row or column width should be related to ease of reading and logical. In some cases, it is easier to read two lines of text and in come cases it is easier to have one line of text in a wide column. In the example, two lines of text are needed for the title of the table. That makes sense since none of the characteristics' names are very long.

The final rule of thumb is that units need to be included in the table. Notice in the example table that in all cases the units are provided. In this case, that means years or years old are the units but units are whatever was reported.

Summary

Tables are a common method for epidemiologists to present data. Using tabular format often simplifies the data such that readers can understand the material. Several rules of thumb have been developed in displaying data. These rules of thumb allow readers of epidemiological research to understand complex data in a logical and clear manner.

Concept Reinforcement

1. What does a subordinate position of data tell the reader?

2. Characteristics tables are typically Table 1 in most epidemiological research articles. Why is that?

3. How many lines would it take to write out the data presented in the example? Based on that guess, what is another advantage of using tables that was not described in the text.

Chapter 29 - Graphs and Charts

Chapter Objectives

- List the types of graphs and charts
- Discuss the pros and cons of the different types of graphs and charts
- State the optimal choice for each type of chart

It is often easier to understand study results when these data are presented graphically rather than in a narrative format. Graphs can also be easier to understand than tables. When looking at most types of graphs make sure to pay attention to the horizontal (x-axis) and vertical (y-axis) axis' scale. Occasionally there will be a scale on both the left and right side of the vertical axes.

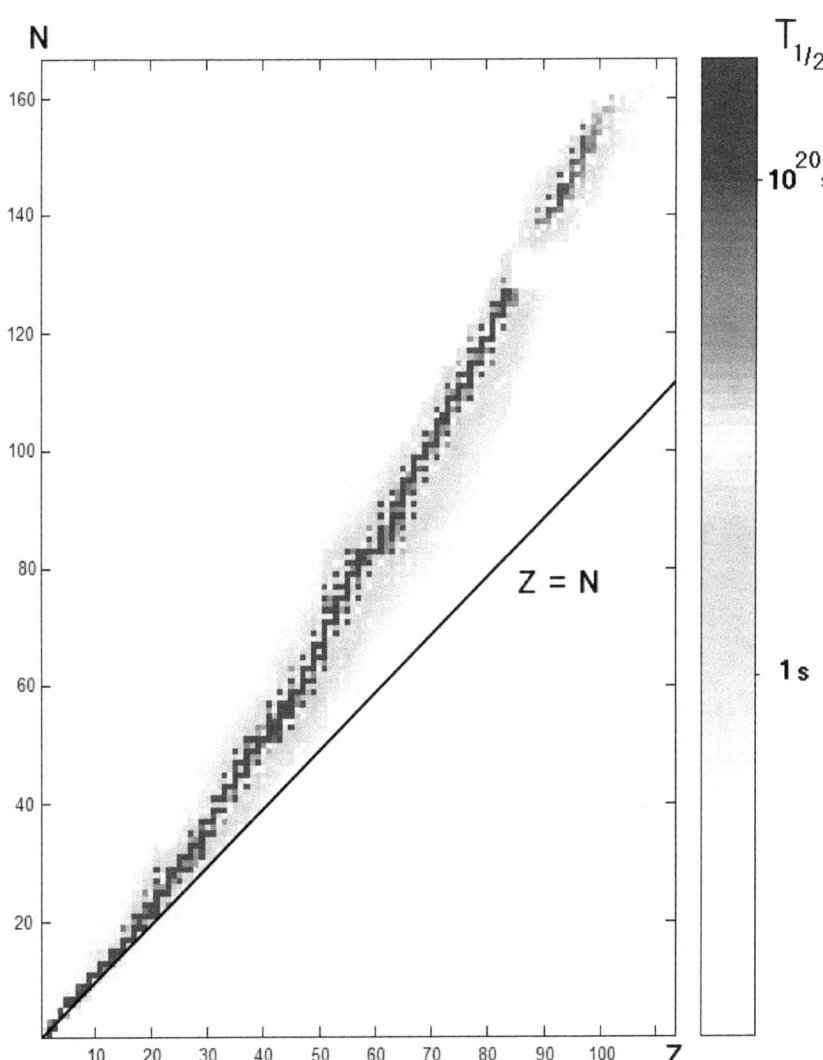

Case Study Description

The following topic is used as an example for all but one of the charts shown in this lesson. Asthma is a chronic respiratory disease that obstructs the airway due to inflammation of the bronchial tubes. This inflammation causes the bronchial tubes to swell. The swelling narrows the airway and makes breathing difficult. An asthma attack can lead to death. Asthma is the leading cause of school absenteeism from chronic conditions. It is also the leading cause of hospitalizations for children under the age of 15 in the US. For those with Medicaid, approximately 25% of all children with asthma will make at least one ER visit a year. The New York City Department of Health and Mental Hygiene's Childhood Asthma Initiative is a public health effort to reduce asthma morbidity among children 0-18 years of age.

Charts (also known as diagrams)

The graphical chart provides a visual display of data that would normally be represented in a table format. Ideally, a chart displays the result in a more reader-friendly format than a table or text such that the idea is more easily conveyed. Presenting data in the format of a chart should allow the reader to quickly grasp what the data mean.

A chart has 3 basic components: labeling that defines the data (title, axis labels, legend), scale (x and y axis range), graphical elements (bars, lines, points).

Bar Chart (Histogram)

Bar charts are one of the most popular types of charts. This chart often displays relation between one or more categorical variables with one or more quantitative variables represented by the length of the bars. The categories are usually on the x-axis (horizontal axis). More than one set of data mandates the use of a legend.

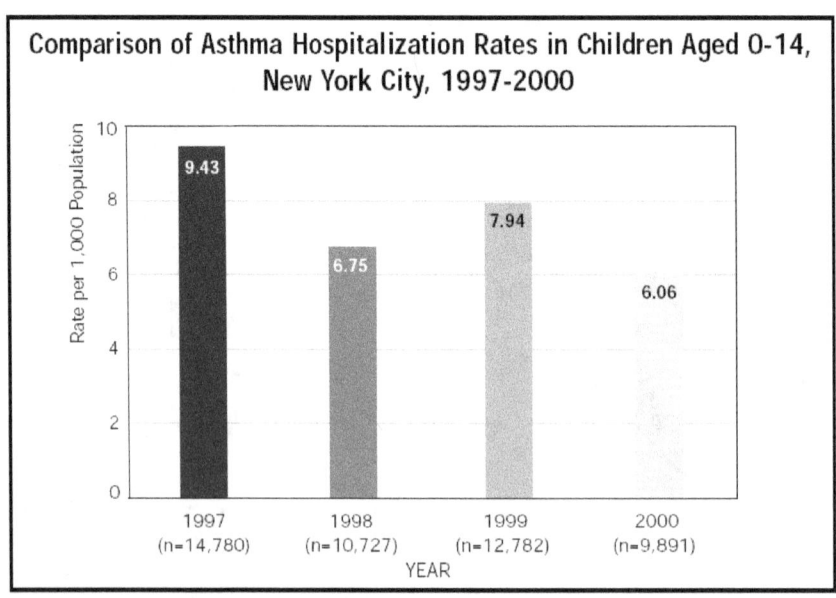

Comparison of asthma hospitalization rates in children aged 0-14, NYC, 1997-2000

In this example, not only are bars used to show the relative magnitude of the hospitalization rates by year, but the color scheme is graduated from dark (highest rate) to light (lowest rate).

It is recommended that no more than seven numbers are included on the x-axis scale. For fewer than five bars, consider using data labels of each bar instead of y-axis scale. This is shown above. If more than 8-10 categories, use a "rotated bar chart" which means the categories are displayed on the y-axis and the values are on the x-axis. This is shown below. Ideally, the data should be sorted on significant variable. (This was not done in the example below.)

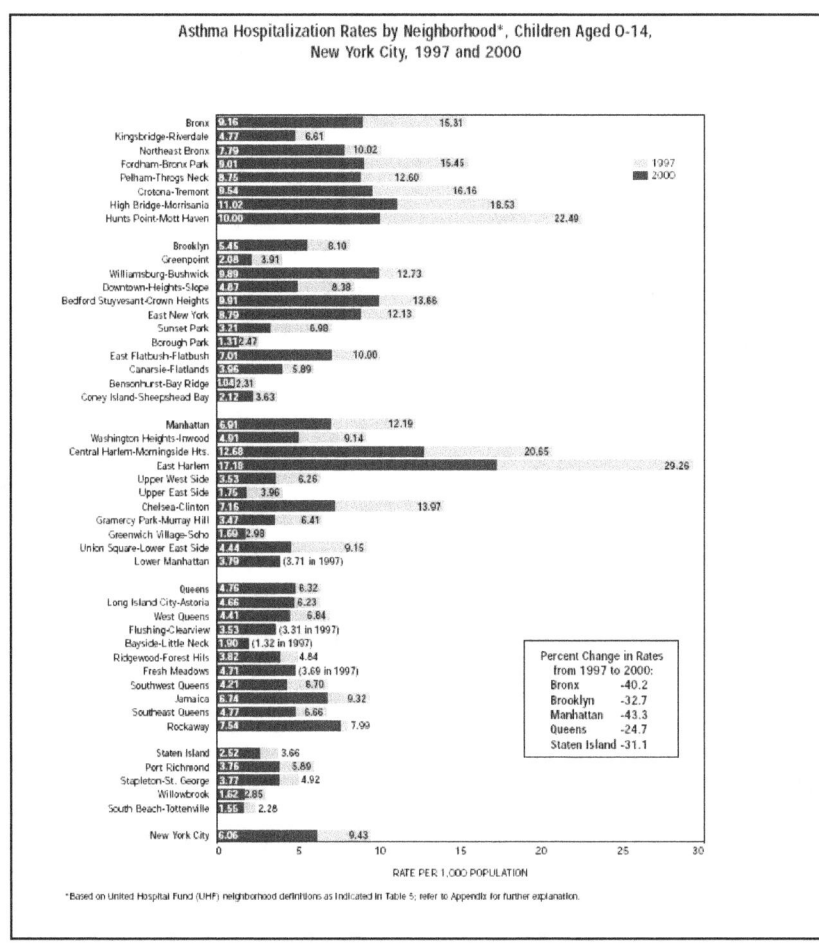

Asthma hospitalization rates by neighborhood in NYC

The legend should be placed either inside the plot area or horizontally under the chart title, not outside of the plot area. This minimizes the size of the area given to displaying these data.

Stacked bar charts have limited use and are rarely an effective display of data. These work best when showing primary comparisons across series among categories.

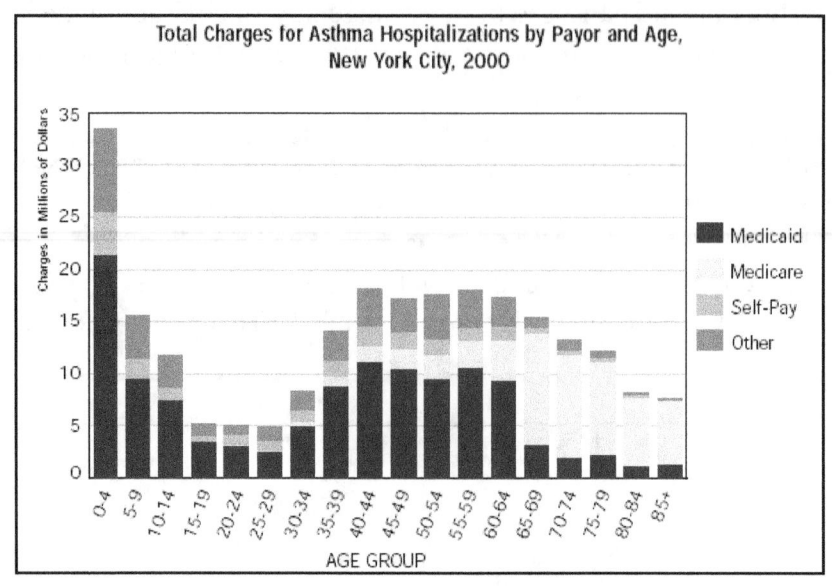

Total charges for asthma hospitalization by payer and age, NYC, 2000

Although it seems to be visually interesting, rarely is a 3-d bar chart the best choice in unambiguously displaying data and therefore should be avoided.

Line Chart

Line charts should only be used when a period of time is involved. This type of chart is ideal for showing trends. The time dimension is almost always shown on the x-axis from left to right. Be careful of scaling effect when more than one variable is presented on a chart. Usually the variable with the larger scale will appear to have a greater degree of variation and the smaller scale when appear more "flat," even though the percent change may be the same. When several time series are presented in the same chart using black and white print, mixing solid, dotted and dashed lines for each variable can help distinguish between them.

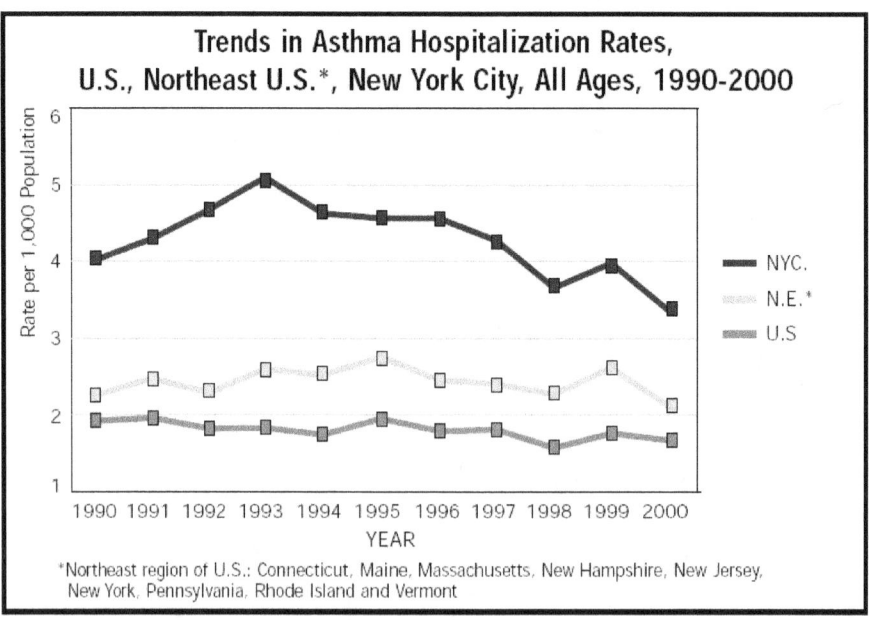

Trends in asthma hospitalization rates, US Northeast US, NYC

Pie Chart

Of all types of charts, pie charts should be avoided since they lack clarity. In addition, 3-d pie charts are worse than 2-d pie charts because adding the "depth" dimension adds no information. It seems that the 3-d pie chart is used for aesthetic purposes not to accurately and efficiently display information. If one insists on using a pie chart, then these should only be used for displaying proportions and only if the data add up to some meaningful total.

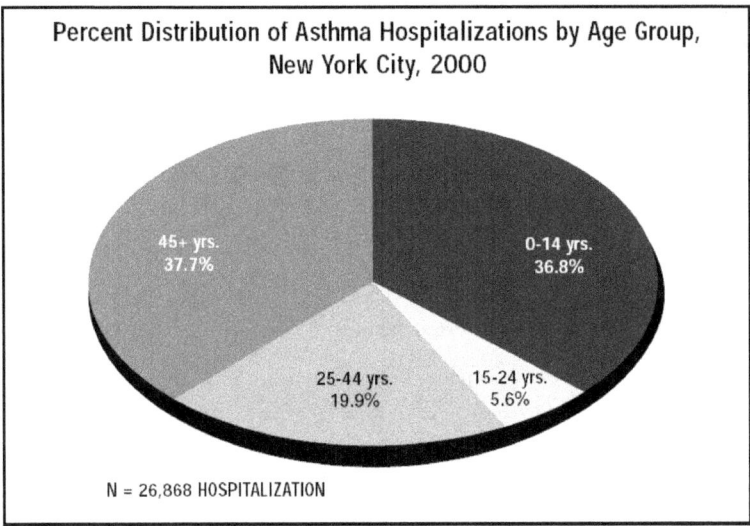

Percent distribution of asthma hospitalizations by age group, NYC, 2000

Boxplots

Boxplots display distribution and interval-level variables. The median and four quartiles are displayed. Boxplots are best used for comparing the distribution of the same variable for two or more groups or two or more time points. Boxplots are also effective in displaying a single case compared to a large number of other cases.

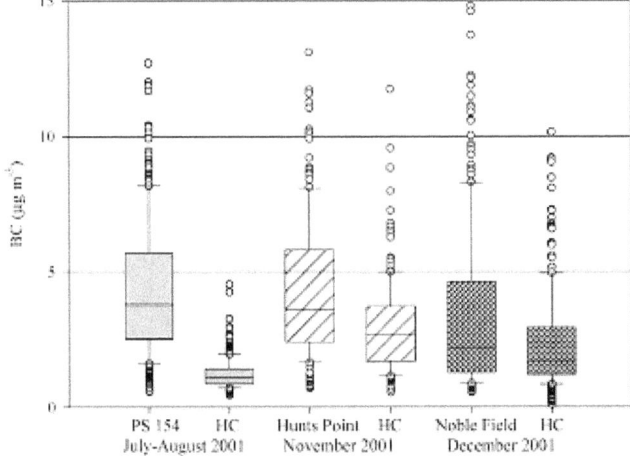

Figure. Concurrent hourly arithmetic mean BC (black carbon) concentration (μgm-3) measured at three South Bronx sites and Hunter College (HC). Line in the box is a median, box size 25th -75th percentile. Circles are outliers (measurements outside the 10th and 90th percentile).

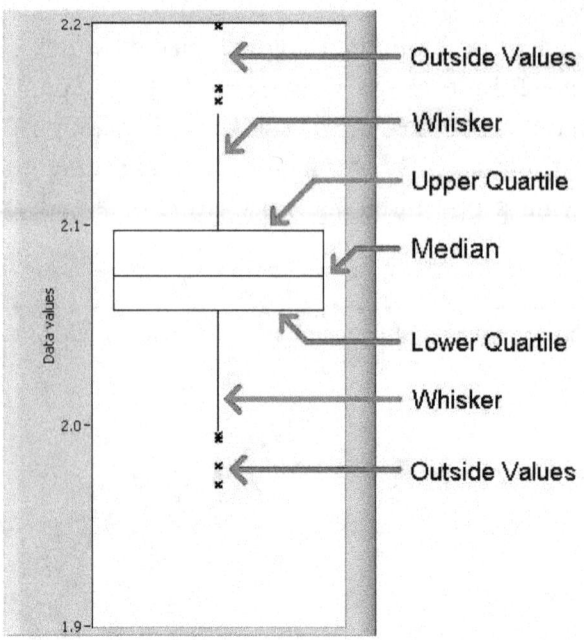

Parts of a box plot

Summary

Epidemiology is rich in data. Displaying these data in such a manner that allows for easy understanding is a skill that is honed in epidemiology. The use of tables and charts is one of the most common means by which epidemiologist report results since these graphics allow for a considerable amount of data to be shared in an organized manner. By describing the data through graphics, a clear presentation of data is likely to result. A clear presentation improves communication of important research findings.

Concept Reinforcement

1. Explain the difference between a histogram and a line chart.

2. Discuss why pie charts are usually avoided when presenting epidemiologic data.

3. List the components of a box plot and describe when box plots are useful in presenting information

Chapter 30 - Person, Time, and Place

Chapter Objectives

- Describe the component of person
- Describe the component of time
- Describe the component of place

There are three primary components of a descriptive epidemiologic study: person, time and place. These are essential when documenting an epidemiologic outbreak and monitoring the spread of a disease. Person refers to the individuals of interest. These may be people who have an exposure, develop a disease, or are otherwise of interest to the epidemiologist. Each person who develops a disease or has an exposure is a case. Time refers to the time frame over which the disease or illness occur. Place is the location of the participants. Depending on the purpose of a study, all three of these pieces of information may need to be collected.

Components of Person

Of the three fundamental components of descriptive epidemiology, describing participants has received the most attention. Below are a few common characteristics.

Age

Several characteristics are important to collect about participants. Age is important. The human biological clock phenomenon means that as a person ages s/he becomes more vulnerable to illness. Lifestyle also influences some chronic diseases, such as Type II diabetes.

The United States is graying. This means the number of people over 65 years old is increasing. About 35 million Americans are 65 years old or more in mid 2000s. By 2030, the number is projected to double. With this phenomena, more epidemiological studies will be needed on the topic of "retirement syndrome," the bereavement process, and other health related issues among older adults.

Sex and Race

Other characteristics are sex and race. Predictors of diseases may vary by both of these characteristics. Further, lifestyle choices may also be different according to sex or race. Therefore, information about these two characteristics is important to collect.

Marital Status

Marital status is generally categorized as single or never married, married or living with a partner, separated, divorced and widowed. The married category has changed over time. In the 1950s, the term "living with a partner" would not have appeared on a survey since there was social sigma associated with this situation. However, these days that social stigma is significantly reduced and about 11 million people reported that they were living with an unmarried partner in the U.S. Census.

Epidemiological studies have shown that married couples have lower morbidity and mortality, especially men. People who have never married are less likely to be overweight whereas being married is linked to obesity, especially for men.

What is it about being married that confers protection against some diseases? One protective hypothesis is that healthier people are more likely to get married and stay married. Another protective hypothesis is that the state of marriage makes a positive contribution to health, including lifestyle choices or financial wellbeing.

Socioeconomic Status

The financial well being of people has been noted since the beginning of time. It is well known that wealth is associated with health. Impoverished people have higher death rates than wealthy people. The advantage of social class is graduated so that each change in social class confer improved health. These statistics are at the group level. This means that with any class of people there will be some who die young or become severely ill. However, as a group the patterns holds regarding increased social position linked with better health.

Components of Place

Another component of descriptive epidemiology is gathering data about place. It is well known that geographical variation is seen on the global scale.

Among Counties Variation

Both chronic diseases such as cancer and heart disease and infectious diseases such as malaria and cholera vary by county. Life expectancy reflects geographic variations in the illnesses and diseases faced by each county.

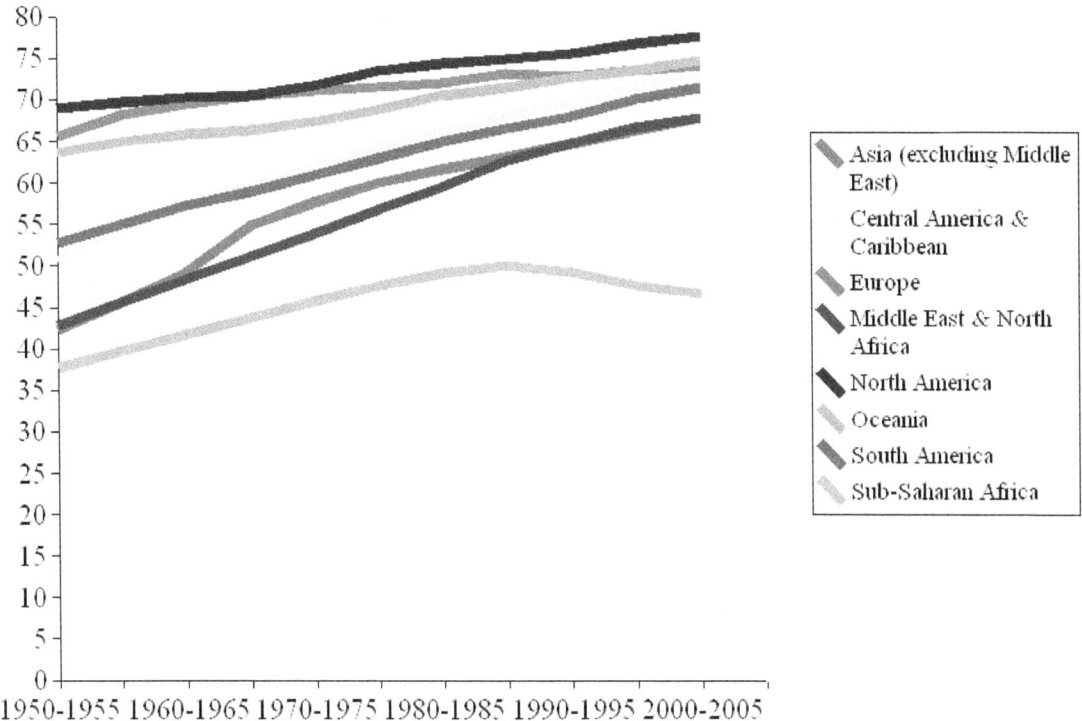

Comparison of life expectancy in 2000 and 2025 by country

Within Country Geographic Variation

Within the United States, there is considerable geographic variation in climate, environmental pollution, and clustering of different types of people.

Urban and Rural Differences

Living in the city or country is associated with different exposures. Obviously, city people live in more crowded conditions where the spread of infectious diseases occurs more readily. People living in agricultural rural areas are more likely to be exposed to pesticides.

Regional Variations

Patterns of illness or diseases can also be observed in larger regions of the country. For example AIDS rates are higher in the Northeast than other regions of the United States and this pattern has remained constant over time. The south leads the county in obesity. More people in the south are obese than in other regions of the county.

Components of Time

The final component of descriptive epidemiology is gathering data about time. The time component associated with a disease is known as temporal aspect of disease. In some cases examining the time dimension can help understand the disease process.

Cyclic Fluctuations

> **Fluctuation**
> An increase or decrease in the number of cases over time.

Many cases of seasonal trends in health conditions are observed. For example birth rates increase in early summer. Feeling depressed also shows an increase in early summer. Cyclic fluctuation can occur within a year as shown with birth data and depressive symptoms. It can also occur within decades. For example, pneumonia-influenza shows periodic epidemics every few years.

Many disease that show cyclic flucutations related to changes in lifestyle behaviors. For example, an increase in Malaria can not occur in winter when the mosquito cannot live.

Secular Time Trends

Secular time trends means that changes in the frequency of a disease is gradual and takes a long period of time. For example, lung cancer has increased in women with the change in smoking behavior of women. In the mid 1990s few women smoked. With the increase in smoking behavior by women in the late 1990s, the rate of lung cancer has increased.

Summary

Person, place and time are important characteristics of the participants. Depending on the epidemiological study, the importance of each of these may vary. Sometimes, knowing the location of a person does not add any useful information to the study. The same is also true for the time component and some of the characteristics of the person. Epidemiologists always give thoughtful consideration of each of these three characteristics when designing their studies.

Concept Reinforcements

1. What could a high rate of a disease in a geographic area suggest to the researcher?

2. What do you think is the most important characteristic of a country related to life expectancy?

3. Do you think there is any disease or health condition that shows no international variation? If no, explain; if yes, which one and explain.

Chapter 31 - Case-control Study Design

Chapter Objectives

- Explain the concept of counterfactual
- Compare the three types of causality
- Describe the Bradford Hill Criteria

Epidemiology is the study population health. Epidemiological researchers use various measurements determine exposures. A key concept in determining exposures is causality.

Determining Causality

Epidemiologic researchers prefer to be able to determine the *cause* of the illness, disease, injury, or health outcome. However, it is not possible to determine the cause with 100% confidence for a couple of basic reasons. One reason is that it is unethical to expose people to a known health risk to study the effects of that exposure. In the current political climate, extraordinary efforts have been instituted to protect study participants. The second reason it is difficult to determine cause that humans are biologically complicated creatures unique individual experiences. Because of the variety of experience and the level of biological complexity, teasing out the cause-effect path is daunting, to say the least.

No two people are alike. Even if a researcher takes into account as many experiences and exposures as humanly possible, there will still be an uncountable number of experiences and exposures that differ between any two people. Dr. Kenneth Rothman uses the counterfactual ideal to explain the difficulty of determining causal relationships. In an ideal comparison, a person will be compared to him or herself. In one state, the person is not exposed and in the other state the person is exposed to whatever is begin tested. If this could happen, researchers would be able to determine the effect of exposure because the exposure would really be the only difference between the two situations. However, we do not have two identities or parallel existences. Consequently, this situation is called **counterfactual**.

Another facet of the counterfactual situation described above is the necessity of having the exposed and unexposed experiences happen simultaneously so that a time dimension does not influence the study results. The closest that an epidemiologic study comes to this possibility is the **crossover design**. In this design, the participant is randomly placed in either the treatment or control group. After a certain amount of time, the participants switch groups. In other words, the treatment groups become the control group and visa versa. This design comes close to achieving a counterfactual comparison. However, the design falls short because a person can only be in one study group at a time. The time component may affect the study results since the passage of time may introduce different factors other than the treatment.

> **Crossover Design**
>
> Participants assume both the treatment and control experience.
>
> Participants are randomly assigned to one or the other group, first.
>
> The subjects act as their own controls.

> **Counterfactual**
>
> Contrary to the facts.
>
> A condition which cannot be fulfilled.

To reiterate, in a counterfactual study, each exposed participant would be compared to his/her unexposed self while facing simultaneous experiences. The number of exposed participants who develop the disease would be compared to the number of unexposed participants who develop the disease. The difference would indicate the effect of the exposure. For example, in a group of 100, let's say we found 1 in 4 (25% exposed participants developed the disease and of this same counterfactual group of 100 people, 1 in 10 (10% unexposed participants developed the disease. The causal effect of the exposure would be 15% (25%–10% = 15%. The causal effects of the exposure is the percent of people who were exposed to the variable and who developed the disease minus the group of people who were NOT exposed to the variable and developed the disease. The difference is disease incidence between these two groups is the causal effect.

Since the ideal of a counterfactual experience cannot occur, epidemiologists carefully design their studies to minimize the differences between the comparison groups. The goal is to find an unexposed population that reflects a counterfactual situation as closely as possible. Suppose we use the same examples as above and, instead of having a counterfactual group, we compare our exposed group to another group of people who were unexposed. The gold standard for researchers is for the unexposed group to simulate all the important experiences of the exposed group. Using the same disease rates as above, a lack of a true counterfactual experience precludes the researcher from being 100% sure that the 15% difference between the two groups is absolutely due to the exposure. The solution that epidemiologist use as guidelines to determining a causal link are the Bradford-Hill criteria, which we will discuss later in this chapter.

Causal Relation

Let's look a little closer at the task of identifying causal relation in scientific research. Causality can be categorized into three fundamental types in order to decreasing strength or sufficiency as a cause. They are 1 a **sufficient cause**, 2 a **necessary cause**, and 3 a **risk factor**.

Sufficient cause is rarely observed in epidemiology. The factor must be present before the disease *and* it always predicts the occurrence of the disease. Genetic abnormalities are the best example of this type of causality.

A **necessary cause** often involves an external exposure. This factor must be present for the disease to develop but not everyone who is exposed to this factor will develop the disease or illness. Infectious diseases are good examples of necessary cause. For example, exposure to the *tubercle bacillus* may result in the person developing tuberculosis. However, some people such as Mary Mallon, also known as Typhoid Mary, are carriers of the disease but do not suffer any symptoms.

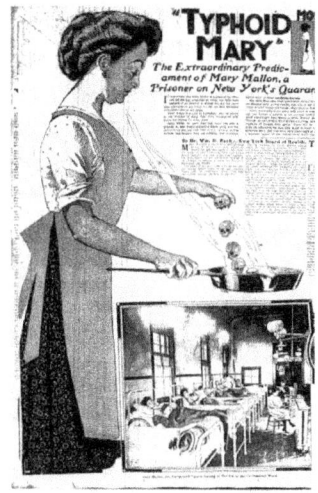

Mary Mallon, also known as Typhoid Mary, carried the disease typhoid and infected people even though she did not get sick from the disease.

The weakest causal type is a **risk factor**. When the factor is present, the probability of the disease increases. A risk factor is neither a necessary or sufficient cause of the disease. Smoking is a classic risk factor for lung cancer. It is not a sufficient cause since some people who never smoke are diagnosed with lung cancer. In other words, smoking does NOT always predict the occurrence of lung cancer therefore it cannot be classified as a sufficient or necessary causal agent. However, smoking is considered a very strong risk factor for lung cancer. For heavy male smokers, the probability of developing lung cancer is 20 times higher compared to non-smoking men.

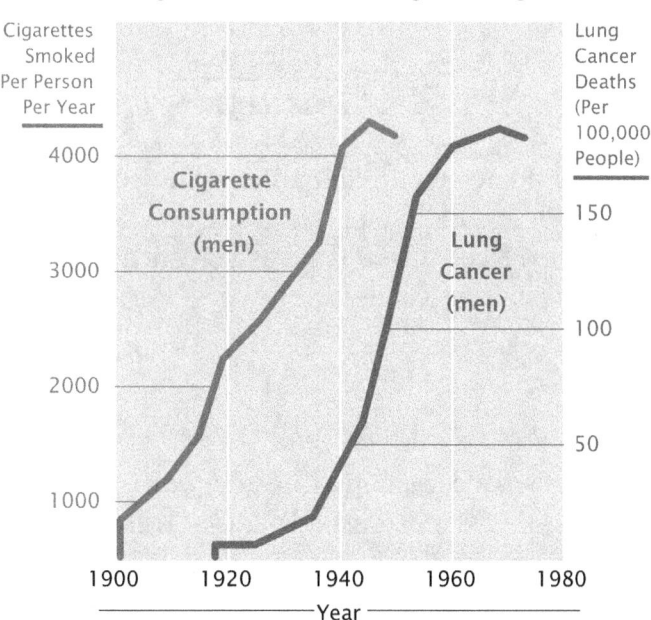

Correlation between smoking and lung cancer in US males, showing a 20-year time lag between increased smoking rates and increased incidence of lung cancer

Image courtesy of the National Institutes of Health

The debate about whether or not smoking causes lung cancer can be considered in light of these definitions. Often the tobacco company's spokesperson will use the definition of sufficient or necessary cause when speaking about the lack of evidence that smoking cigarettes causes lung cancer. In contrast, the majority of researchers feel confident saying smoking causes lung cancer, even though it is the weakest type of causality.

Risk

The word **risk** is commonly used in epidemiology and is often applied to individuals. Risk is interchangeable with the term probability. The risk of an individual being diagnosed with an illness is the same as the probability of an individual being diagnosed with an illness. However, except for the on-lines tools that allow individuals to determine his/her particular risk based on certain medical histories and lifestyle behaviors, it is common to study the risk of disease at the population level. In this case, the proportion of people who developed the disease during a specified period of time represents the risk of the disease in the population during the specified time frame.

The risk of a specified population is equal to	The number of individuals who were diagnosed with the disease during a specified time period divided by
	The total number of individuals in the specific population

Before continuing, let's review basic math terminology for fractions. The top number is known as the numerator and the bottom number is known as the denominator.

$$Fraction = \frac{Numerator}{Denominator}$$

Typically, figuring out the numerator in a study is quite straightforward. However, the denominator is much trickier and the use of the wrong population in the denominator will result in useless study results. Keep this in mind as you are designing epidemiological experiments and analyzing the data you collect.

The Bradford Hill Criteria

The public wants to know "what caused my disease." To help answer that question from epidemiologic study results, in 1965 Sir Austin Bradford Hill described the nine conditions needed to establish a causal relationship.

Nine Conditions Required to Establish a Causal Relationship:

- **Strength of association**—the relationship must be clear as defined by the size of the association measured by appropriate statistical tests. For example, the more highly correlated hypertension is with a high sodium diet, the stronger is the relation between sodium and hypertension.

- **Consistency**—observation of the association must be repeatable in different populations at different times and in different settings.

- **Temporality**—the exposure must always precede the outcome (disease) in time.

- **Plausibility**—the explanation must make sense biologically. However, studies that disagree with established understanding of biological processes may force a re-evaluation of accepted beliefs.

- **Dose**-response relationship—increasing amount of exposure increases the risk.

- **Specificity** –a single cause produces a specific effect. This is considered to be the weakest criteria. Absence of specificity in no way negates a causal relationship.

- **Coherence** – explanation should coincide with natural history and biology of the disease.

- **Experiment**– any related research that is based on experiments.

- **Analogy** – sometimes a commonly accepted phenomenon in one area can be applied to another area.

Concept Extension: Institutional Review Boards

The Research Act of 1974 defined Institutional Review Boards (IRBs). IRBs are independent ethics committees that have been formally designated to approve, monitor, and review biomedical and behavioral research involving humans. The purpose of IRBs is to protect the rights and welfare of the study participants. In the United States, the U.S. Food and Drug Administration and the Department of Health and Human Services' regulations have empowered IRBs to approve, require modifications, and/or disapprove research. The reason that IRBs were developed was because of research abuses earlier in the 20th century.

One well-known case of research abuse occurred during WWII in which Nazi physicians performed experiments on prisoners of war. Some of these abuses were exposed during the Nuremberg Trials.

In the United States, the Tuskegee Syphilis Study was an unethical and scientifically unjustifiable project. In 1932, the Public Health Service and the Tuskegee Institute began a project to study the natural course of syphilis. The study enrolled poor, illiterate black men from rural Alabama (399 with syphilis and 201 without syphilis). There was no participant's informed consent. In fact, the participants were deceived about the study. Those with syphilis did not receive proper treatment when penicillin became available and the accepted treatment.

Protection of human subjects' definition

Human subject means a living individual about whom an investigator (whether professional or student) conducting research obtains (1) data through intervention or interaction with the individual, or (2) identifiable private information.

Intervention includes both physical procedures by which data are gathered (for example, a blood draw) and manipulations of the subject or the subject's environment that are performed for research purposes.

Interaction includes communication or interpersonal contact between investigator and subject.

Private information includes information about behavior that occurs in a context in which an individual can reasonably expect that no observation or recording is taking place, and information which has been provided for specific purposes by an individual and which the individual can reasonably expect will not be made public (for example, a medical record). Private information must be individually identifiable (i.e. the identity of the subject is obvious or may readily be ascertained by the investigator or associated with the information) in order for obtaining the information to constitute research involving human subjects.

Research means a systematic investigation, including research development, testing and evaluation, designed to develop or contribute to generalizable knowledge. Activities that meet this definition constitute research for purposes of this policy, whether or not they are conducted or supported under a program that is considered research for other purposes (for example, some demonstration and service programs may include research activities).

Minimal risk means that the probability and magnitude of harm or discomfort anticipated in the research are not greater in and of themselves than those ordinarily encountered in daily life or during the performance of routine physical or psychological examinations or tests.

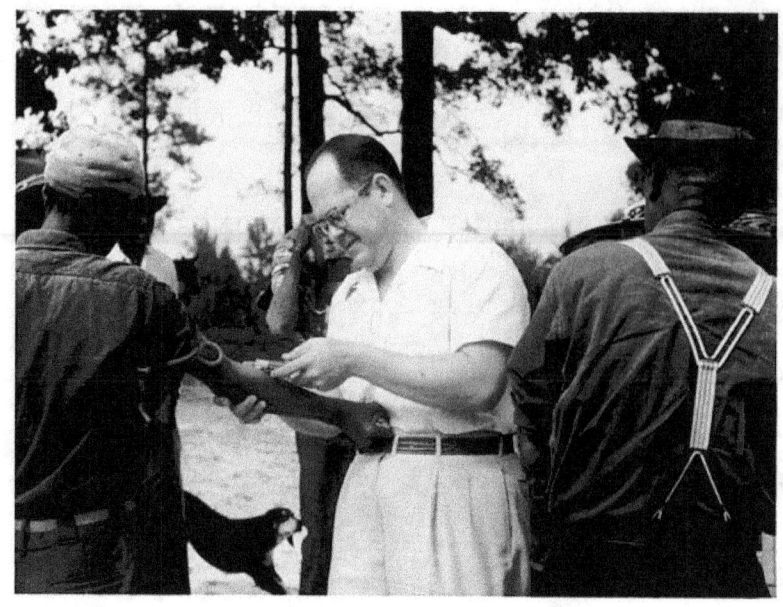

Examination, Tuskegee study

Image courtesy of the National Archives and Records Administration, US Government

The IRB (institutional review board) at almost all institutions, such as universities and hospitals that engage in human research, review research projects that involve humans to ensure that ethical standards outlined by the Federal Policy for the Protection of Human Subjects (45 CFR (Code of Federal Regulations) 46) are adhered to in conducting research using human subjects.

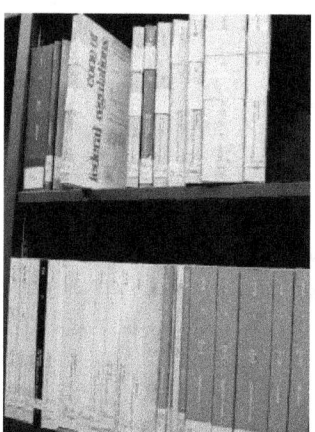

Code of Federal Regulations, seen at the Mid-Manhattan Library. Editions of Title 3, on the President, are kept on archive. Notice that for the first year of each new presidency, the volume is thicker.

Code of Federal Regulations, Title 45: Public Welfare, Department of Health and Human Services, Part 46: Protection of Human Subjects (45 CFR 46)

Who must follow this policy?

Any research conducted or supported by any federal agency or department. There are also some other types of research that must comply but we won't go into the details of those.

46.116: General requirements for informed consent

No investigator may involve a human being as a subject in research covered by this policy unless the investigator has obtained the legally effective *informed consent* of the subject or the subject's legally authorized representative.

46.116a: Basic elements mandated to be included in the consent form

(1) A statement that the study involves research, an explanation of the purposes of the research and the expected duration of the subject's participation, a description of the procedures to be followed, and identification of any procedures which are experimental;

(2) A description of any reasonably foreseeable risks or discomforts to the subject;

(3) A description of any benefits to the subject or to others which may reasonably be expected from the research;

(4) A disclosure of appropriate alternative procedures or courses of treatment, if any, that might be advantageous to the subject;

(5) A statement describing the extent, if any, to which confidentiality of records identifying the subject will be maintained;

(6) For research involving more than minimal risk, an explanation as to whether any compensation and an explanation as to whether any medical treatments are available if injury occurs and, if so, what they consist of, or where further information may be obtained;

(7) An explanation of whom to contact for answers to pertinent questions about the research and research subjects' rights, and whom to contact in the event of a research-related injury to the subject; and

(8) A statement that participation is voluntary, refusal to participate will involve no penalty or loss of benefits to which the subject is otherwise entitled, and the subject may discontinue participation at any time without penalty or loss of benefits to which the subject is otherwise entitled.

Who is exempt from having to obtain IRB approval? 46.101b

1) Research conducted in established or commonly accepted educational settings, involving normal educational practices, such as (i) research on regular and special education instructional strategies, or (ii) research on the effectiveness of or the comparison among instructional techniques, curricula, or classroom management methods.

(2) Research involving the use of educational tests (cognitive, diagnostic, aptitude, achievement), survey procedures, interview procedures or observation of public behavior, unless: (i) information obtained is recorded in such a manner that human subjects can be identified, directly or through identifiers linked to the subjects; and (ii) any disclosure of the human subjects' responses outside the research could reasonably place the subjects at risk of criminal or civil liability or be damaging to the subjects' financial standing, employability, or reputation.

(3) Research involving the use of educational tests (cognitive, diagnostic, aptitude, achievement), survey procedures, interview procedures, or observation of public behavior that is not exempt under paragraph (b)(2) of this section, if: (i) the human subjects are elected or appointed public officials or candidates for public office; or (ii) federal statute(s) require(s) without exception that the confidentiality of the personally identifiable information will be maintained throughout the research and thereafter.

(4) Research involving the collection or study of existing data, documents, records, pathological specimens, or diagnostic specimens, if these sources are publicly available or if the information is recorded by the investigator in such a manner that subjects cannot be identified, directly or through identifiers linked to the subjects.

(5) Research and demonstration projects which are conducted by or subject to the approval of department or agency heads, and which are designed to study, evaluate, or otherwise examine: (i) Public benefit or service programs; (ii) procedures for obtaining benefits or services under those programs; (iii) possible changes in or alternatives to those programs or procedures; or (iv) possible changes in methods or levels of payment for benefits or services under those programs.

(6) Taste and food quality evaluation and consumer acceptance studies, (i) if wholesome foods without additives are consumed or (ii) if a food is consumed that contains a food ingredient at or below the level and for a use found to be safe, or agricultural chemical or environmental contaminant at or below the level found to be safe, by the Food and Drug Administration or approved by the Environmental Protection Agency or the Food Safety and Inspection Service of the U.S. Department of Agriculture.

Complying with all the elements in this policy is time consuming for researchers and it typically takes 2-6 months to obtain IRB approval from their institution. The IRB has dozens of research projects to review at each meeting. If they have any questions about a particular project, they generate a letter listing their questions, directives or concerns. The researcher has to respond to every item in the letter and resubmit the application to the IRB. The application is put into queue again. This back and forth exchange can happen numerous times.

Many institutional IRBs meet every two weeks. So the cycle on any formal communication is at best one month. Probably the biggest area of back and forth communication is the elements of the consent letter and/or introductory letter. There is no template for this and therefore every submission has the potential to generate new or different concerns from the IRB, even for essentially identical studies.

A large literature exists that describes people's perception of risk and how they communicate using probability terms. For example, people who have had a health problem are more likely to rate it higher on the probability scale than someone without the experience. Events that are more common are more likely to be ranked higher than less common events. Memorable experiences are more likely to rank higher on the probability scale than less memorable experiences. Unfortunately, even though we can describe these and many more differences, there is not a foolproof system we can use to predict how someone will rank the probability so that we could institute a systemic correction to an individual's imprecise risk communication.

Summary

In a perfect world, the researcher would prefer to be able to figure out the causes of injury, illness, and disease. However, they lack a counterfactual model and are left with less than perfect tools to determine the causal factors in diseases. Generally, causal factors are those that can be shown to increase the likelihood of a disease occurrence. Epidemiologists work with three basic forms of causal relationships: necessary cause, sufficient cause and risk factor. In 1965, Sir Austin Bradford Hill described the nine conditions needed to establish a causal relationship. These include strength of association, temporality, consistency, plausibility, dose-response relationship, specificity, coherence, experiment, and analogy.

Concept Reinforcement

1. Explain the concept of counterfactual.

2. List and describe the three types of causality.

3. List and describe the Bradford Hill criteria.

Chapter 32 - Sampling Error and Chance

Chapter Objectives

- Compare random and nonrandom sampling
- Describe simple random sampling
- Define systematic error and random error

Regardless of the source of the data, an important aspect of epidemiology is developing an understanding of these data. In this chapter, we will explore the components of sampling.

Most health research collects data from individuals. Researchers are interested in specific details about individuals, but must also be careful about protecting the privacy of the people in their studies. Oddly, the researcher is very interested in knowing lots of information about an individual but is not interested in the identity of the individual. Except for medical reports, called case study in which a unique medical situations is described and a case series in which several examples of a unique medical situation is described, the individual data is combined and group results are reported.

Population
ALL individuals in a population

Sample
A subset of a population

It is important to know the difference between two terms used in epidemiology: population and sample. A population means ALL individuals. The image below shows a school of fish. The population includes all members of the school. A sample would include a subset of the school of fish. For example, a sample of this school of fish might be five or ten members of the school.

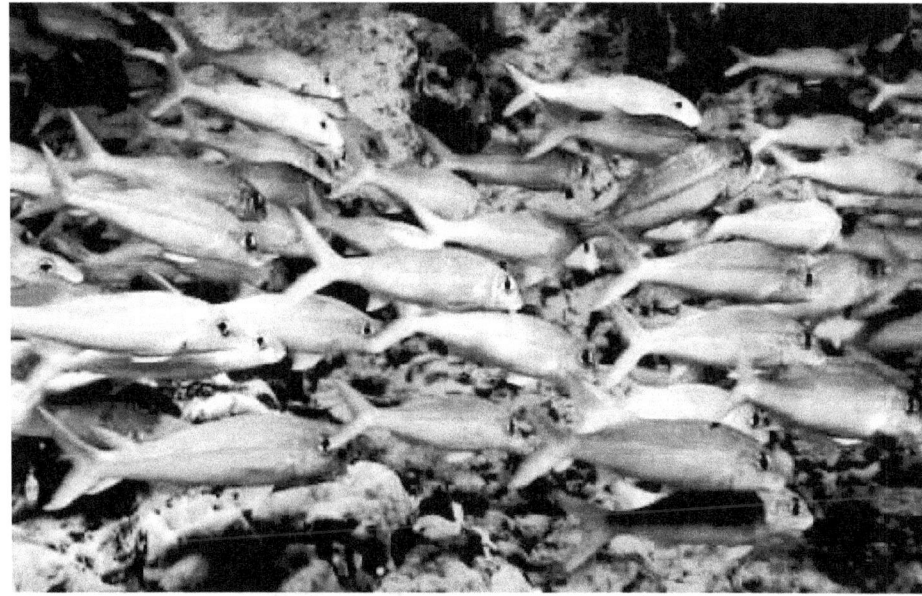

School of yellow-fin goatfish (*Mulloidichthysvanicolensis*)

Image courtesy of the US Government

Simple Random Sample

This is the basic type of probability sampling plan. Every individual in the sampling frame has an equal chance of being selected for the study. A common technique used to select individuals from a list is to use a random digit generator. Each person is assigned a random number. The list is sorted in numerical order using the random digit column. If the researcher wants to approach 416 potential respondents from a list of 1,200 individuals, the sample will consist of the first 416 names on the list after it has been randomized.

Random and Systematic Error

In sampling, the error occurs by the very nature of participant selection, and depends on who was and, more importantly, was not included in the study. Errors can be classified as either systematic or random. Systematic error is nonrandom error in which the values tend to be inaccurate in a particular direction. For example, measuring participants' heights with their shoes on would be a systematic error. Everyone would be slightly taller than if their height was determined without shoes. If participants were measured in bare feet, there would still be random error. Random error means that some of these data would be too high and some would be too low. Random error can occur by chance or lack of knowledge of all relevant factors.

Chance

Many people believe in chance. Chance can play a fundamental role in both biological and physical phenomena. On the other hand, some believe that any situation could be a predicted if all the relevant factors were known. Therefore, we can define random variation as ignorance of all the relevant factors that predict a disease. In the commonly used example of tossing a coin, predicting heads or tails could be determined by applying the physical laws associated with the toss. However, the complexity of the calculation and the lack of necessary information available on the street (such as wind turbulence in the microenvironment) in essence transform this predictable situation into chance or guesswork. Consequently, in epidemiology variation is treated as random until it can be explained, whether the variation is based upon chance or based on insufficient information about relevant factors. All data sampling is subject to random error.

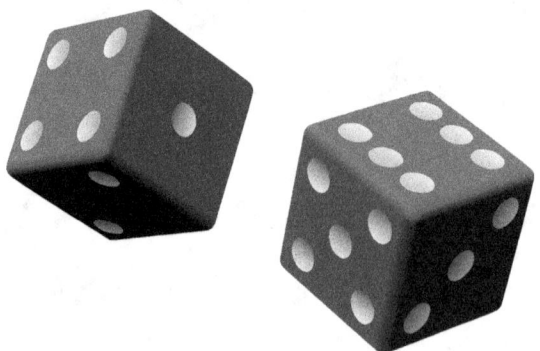

Dice is a game of chance. For example each time you throw the pair of dice, you have only a certain chance of getting a pair of sixes.

Another important component of random variation in epidemiology studies is the process of study subject selection, called sampling. The random variation is known as sampling error. In sampling, the error occurs by the very nature of participant selection, especially who was and, more importantly, was not included in the study. Similarly, measurement error can occur due to the random variation in potential biological experiences of the population. Reducing random error can be accomplished in two ways: increasing sample size or improving the information collected.

Lack of Systematic Error: External Validity

An important component of the study design revolves around the researcher's ability to generalize the findings from the sample of people studied to the appropriate population. Being able to generalize a study to a larger population is called external validity.

Migraine study example

It was once thought by medical professionals that migraines were associated with intelligence. The rationale was that people who used their brains more were more likely to get headache. The parallel was made to those who exercise being more likely to have muscle or joint aches. This theory was debunked in the 70s. It seems this fallacy arose because migraine sufferers that the physicians saw did not represent the population of migraine sufferers. Less intelligent migraine sufferers were much less likely to visit a doctor. This systematic error, the sample studied was systematically more intelligent, led to a lack of external validity in the early migraine studies.

Most studies describe the world in single group studies, for example a survey of students in a school about their dietary habits and their current weight. A study can describe a unique setting where the results only apply to that setting (e.g., students who eat lunch from the salad bar at a school are more likely to be overweight). A study may also describe a typical setting where the results could represent a more general phenomenon (e.g., students who skip breakfast are more likely to be overweight). Choosing the correct sampling process is critical for enhancing external validity.

Lack of Systematic Error: Internal Validity

Validity is the best available approximation of truth of a given population. Internal validity refers to the validity of inferences (cause-effect relation) in studies. Other way internal validity is stated is whether the researcher is measuring what she intends to measure. There are multiple threats to internal validity. One of the threats to internal validity is inconsistency in the comparison groups. Participants bring to the research a myriad of characteristics, including the willingness to participate. If the characteristics of the participants are not similar between the groups, a difficulty arises for the researcher in determining if the differences in the groups are the reason for the study result or has no influence on the study result.

Summary

In data collection when the researcher relies on the participant to provide the information, a difference between fact and reported fact can occur. This is called error. If the error has a pattern to it, it is called systematic error. If a survey has systematic error, then it does not have external validity. External validity means that the results are not believable. Another type of systematic error is internal validity which means the researcher is measurable what is intended to be measured. Maintaining both internal and external validity are necessary parts of a useful study.

Concept Reinforcement

1. Explain the difference between systematic error and random error.

2. In what way would having only volunteers in a study be a problem?

3. Is it possible to ever remove all errors from a study? Explain

Chapter 33 - Sampling Frame

Chapter Objectives

- Define a sampling frame
- Compare the use of lists
- Explain the denominator in the sampling frame

For probability sampling to happen, all individuals of the population of interest have a known, non-zero chance of being selected for the sample. For this to happen, a list of these individuals needs to be compiled. This is known as the sampling frame. There are four basic types of basic probability sampling plans: simple random sampling, systematic sampling, stratified random sampling, and cluster sampling.

> **Sampling Frame**
> A list of the individuals from which a sample will be drawn

Probability

Probability theory tells us that the data gathered from a random sample can be generalized to the population. The measure of this variation is called standard error. Imagine a study of a big city with 10,000,000 inhabitants. Of the ten million inhabitants, 500,000 responded to a survey about whether the city has enough green space. The study results showed that 75% (± 3% which reflects the standard error) of the inhabitants prefer the option of adding more green space. Probability theory tells us that if all ten million inhabitants had been asked, approximately 75% would also have responded by preferring the adding more green space. In general, the larger the sample, the closer the estimate will be to the true population value.

There are four basic types of probabilistic sampling plans: simple random sampling, systematic sampling, stratified random sampling, and cluster sampling. These are described below.

Simple Random Sample

This is the most basic type of probability sampling plan. Every individual in the sampling frame has an equal chance of being selected for the study. A common technique to select individuals from a list is to use a random digit generator. Each person is assigned a random number. The list is sorted in numerical order using the random digit column. The researcher then selects the number of subjects for the study from the list in numerical order.

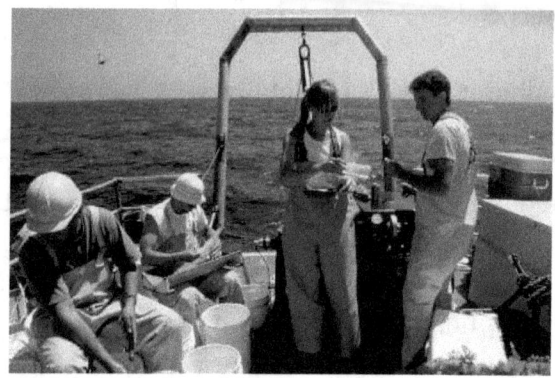

Due to the unique marine environment surrounding the Channel Islands, the Sanctuary is home to a diverse array of marine life, making the region highly valuable to scientific research. The Channel Islands National Marine Sanctuary routinely conducts research to monitor, preserve and protect the sanctuary's rich resources. In 1998, the CINMS participated in a regional monitoring survey of the Southern California Bight coordinated by the Southern California Coastal Water Research Project (SCCWRP). Trawl and sediment samples from randomly selected sights around the islands were collected to measure the distribution and health of the island's marine life.

Image courtesy of the US National Oceanographic and Atmospheric Administration

Systematic Sampling

This is similar to the simple random sample. In this plan, every n^{th} name on the list is selected to be part of the study. For example, using an example of 1,200 students, the list would be divided into 300 groups. To make sure that every student has an equal chance of being selected, for the first group, the selected student would be randomly chosen. After the first student is chosen, the 40th student down the list would be chosen. That means if the number 10 was randomly selected, then student 10 would be chosen, then student number 50 (10+ 40), and so on until the sample is complete.

One advantage of this system is the relative ease of executing the selection process. The randomization procedure only happens once. The major disadvantage to this plan is the possibility that the list may have some type of recurring pattern or cycle. As an illustration, if the researcher uses a list of houses that is a sequential list of houses from block to block and each block has the same number of houses, it could happen that only the corner house on each block is selected. People in these houses might differ from those in the midblock. For example, the corner lot may be the most attractive house on the block and therefore more expensive to rent or own. Another illustration that shows where this type of sampling can go wrong is newspapers. If every seventh paper is chosen, it could happen that this plan selects only Sunday papers. Checking the list for patterns before the sampling plan is implemented is the best method to avoid this problem.

Stratified Random Sampling

The third type of probability sampling is known as stratified random sampling. The population is divided into two or more strata (a particular subgroup within the population, such as male and female) and then either a simple or systematic sampling from each stratum is taken. It is necessary to have an adequate number of potential participants within each stratum to use this strategy. The primary reason researchers prefer a stratifiedrandom sampling plan is that the results may have less variation (less error).

Cluster Sampling

In the other three types of sampling, a sample frame is required. However obtaining a list of potential participations may not be possible. In the above example of high school students, it would be virtually impossible to obtain a list of all high school students in Montana. However, a list of all high schools can be readily obtained. This is known as the cluster. First, a sampling of the cluster is done by either simple or systematic sampling. In this case, a sample is obtained from the list of high schools. After the sample of clusters is chosen, a simple, systematic or stratified random sample of individuals are selected within each school. For this to work, the researchers would need to be able to obtain a list of all high school students in the selected schools. The advantage of this style of sampling is that a sampling frame (complete list of all individuals) is not necessary. The disadvantage is more variation in the study results. Typically, a larger number of individuals are recruited to the study using this sampling plan to offset the larger error in study results.

How Do the Sampling Frame and Samples Relate to One Another?

The sample is a subset of the sampling frame. Remember that the sampling frame is the list of individuals in the population of interest. This may be a small population or a very large population. The sample should be representative of the larger population based on key characteristics, such as socio economic status, gender, race, and other parameters defined by the research team. The statistical methods required to do these analyses often require comparison of the sample to the sampling frame. In math terms, the sample is the numerator of the fraction used to make the comparison and the sampling frame is the denominator.

Summary

The sampling frame is an important component of any epidemiologic study. The sampling frame is the overall population that the researcher wishes to study. This may be a small group of people, such as a classroom full of students, or a very large group, such as the insect population of the Earth. Sampling frames have certain characteristics that may lead the researcher to use different types of sampling techniques. The most basic sampling technique is the simple random sample. Systematic sampling is a relatively simple type of sample where the selection process is based on a pattern, such as every seventh name on a list. Stratified random sampling is slightly more complex because it involves breaking the sampling frame into subgroups, then using random or systematic sampling to draw samples from each subgroup. There are times when a sampling frame cannot be defined. In these situations, it is possible to do cluster sampling. Cluster sampling involves developing a list of the populations, called the cluster. The cluster is sampled, and the samples are further subjected to random, systematic, or stratified sampling methods. Once the data are all collected, the researchers use statistical methods to analyze the results. The sample relates to the sampling frame in the same way the numerator relates to the denominator in a fraction.

Concept Reinforcement

1. List the three types of sampling that use lists and describe how lists are used in each type of sampling.

2. Describe the concept of a sampling frame and why it is important in epidemiology.

3. Explain the denominator in the sampling frame.

Chapter 34 - Confounding and Effect Modifier

Chapter Objectives

- Define confounder
- Define effect modifier
- List examples of confounders

Two terms need to be used correctly when reporting study results: **association** and **cause**. An epidemiologic study is rarely able to demonstrate the cause of a disease. It is typically only able to show associations.

Cause Versus Association

A cause is the reason something happens. There should be two chromosomes in 23 pairs, or a total of 46 chromosomes, in a healthy baby. Trisomy disorders occur when an extra chromosome is made during replication. The specific characteristics of the baby with trisomy disorder are linked to the chromosome. For example, Down syndrome is caused by a chromosome 21 trisomy, the presence of all or part of an extra 21st chromosome. In other words, chromosome trisomy 21 causes Down syndrome.

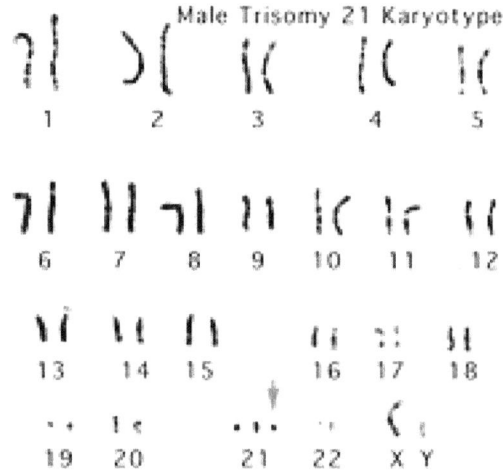

An extra chromosome on chromosome 21

An association is a relation between two variables. In epidemiology, one variable is the risk factor and the other variable is the disease. An association is an indication of the probability of the risk factor being present along with the disease.

If 25% of obese men are rich, 40% of tall men are rich, and being obese does not alter the probability of being rich, then no association exists between weight and financial well being. However, if the prevalence of financial well-being differs in obese men versus tall men, there may be an association between weight and financial well-being. If the weight and height increase together, it is known as a positive association. If the values go in opposite directions, e.g., weight decreases as height increases or visa versa the association is considered negative.

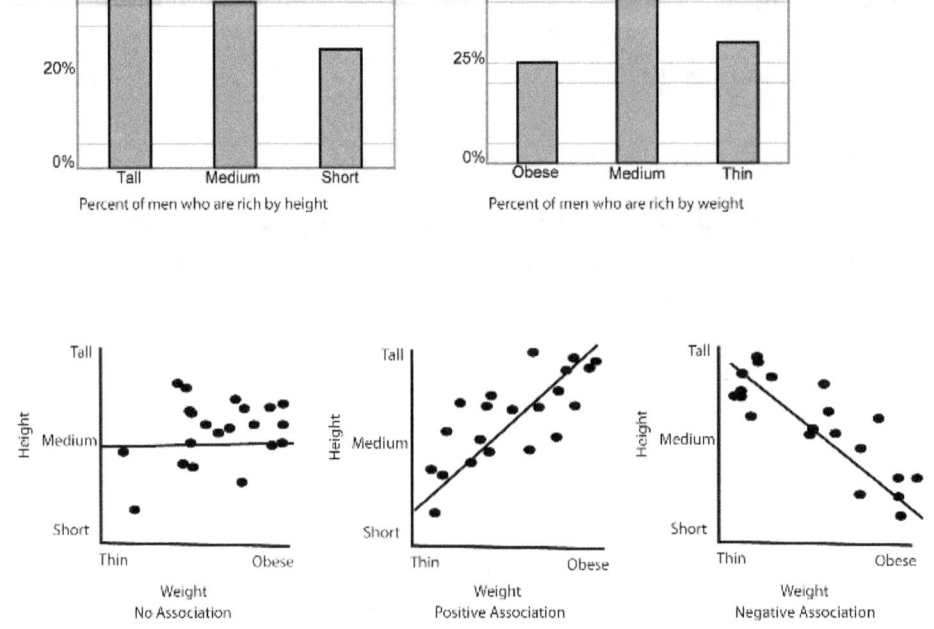

Association between height and weight associated with wealth

Confounders

Is the association real? One common cause of misinterpretation of study results by not distinguishing between confounding and effect modifier. Confounding is when the results suggest a factor as explaining the health outcome but in reality some other factor explains the health outcome. This other factor "goes along" with the first factor. This problem is also known as the influence of the lurking variable (also known as confounder).

Characteristics of Confounders

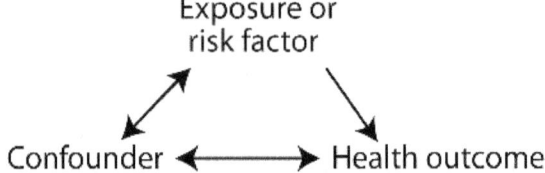

Diagram that shows the association among exposure, confounder and health outcome

When thinking about a confounder the following two points need to be true.

1. The confounder is not on the causal pathway between exposure and disease.
2. The confounder must be associated with both the exposure and the health outcome.

An example might help clarify this concept.

Case Study: Lung Cancer and Bartenders

Several studies using occupational and underlying cause of death data ascertained from death certificates found that bartenders have a high rate of lung cancer. The question that researcher asked was, "What is it about bartenders that may lead to a high lung cancer death rate?"

One possible explanation is that bartenders are more likely to smoke cigarettes. However, it may be that bartenders drink alcohol more than people in other occupations and therefore the reason for the increased lung cancer death rates is directly related to the alcohol consumption of this profession and has nothing to do with cigarette smoking. The hypothesis: there is an association between exposure (cigarette smoking) and a disease (lung cancer). Is alcohol consumption a confounder?

First, we find that cigarette smoking is statistically associated with lung cancer. Cigarette smoking is also associated with alcohol drinking. Therefore, alcohol drinking fulfills one criterion for potential confounding. Alcohol drinking is also associated with lung cancer. Alcohol drinking fulfills the second criterion for potential confounding. However, in the analysis when an adjustment is made for alcohol consumption, the association between drinking alcohol and lung cancer is no longer there. The original association is explained by the fact the more smokers also drink alcohol. The conclusion would be that drinking alcohol is not associated with lung cancer.

Case Study: Down Syndrome and Birth Order

In another example, a study evaluated birth order as a risk factor for increased incidence of Down syndrome.

Below is the table of study results:

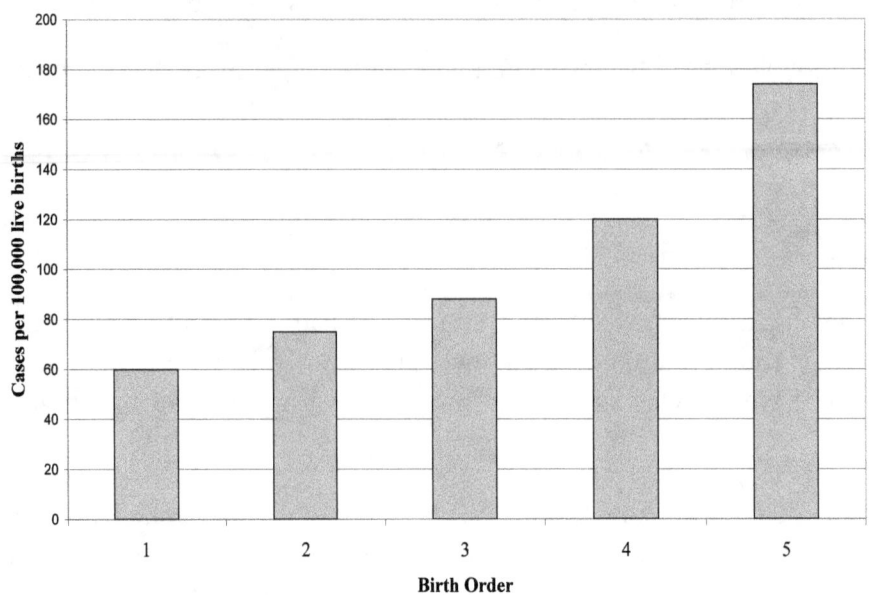

Now let us add another facet to this study.

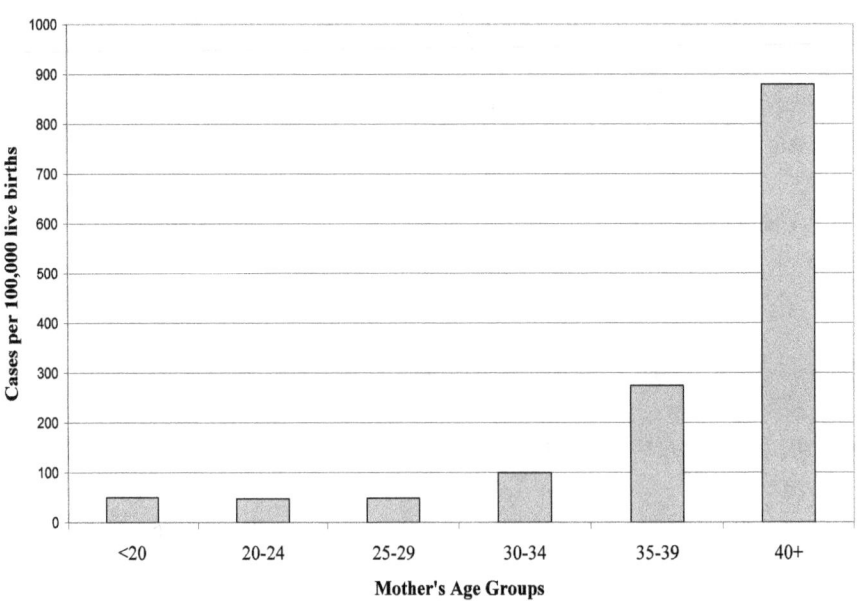

A third factor, which is related to both the exposure (risk factor) and health outcome, and which accounts for some of the observed relationship between the two is a confounder. A confounder is not the result of the exposure. In this case given that we are looking at the association between the child's birth rank (exposure) and Down syndrome (health outcome), is the mother's age a confounder? Given that we are looking at the association between the mother's age (exposure) and Down syndrome (health outcome), is the birth rank a confounder?

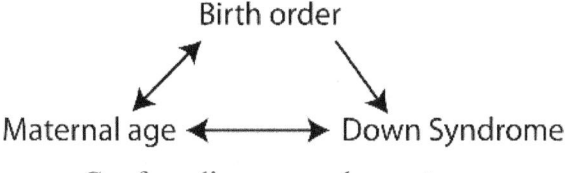
Confounding example, part one

Birth order is associated with maternal age but is not a risk factor in younger mothers.

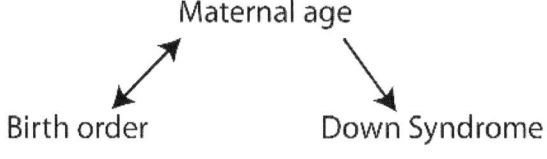
Confounding example, part two

Birth order is associated with maternal age but not a risk factor for Down syndrome in younger mothers. Therefore, it is definitely not a confounder.

Case study: Employment Salaries by Sex

An example in which the lurking variable (confounder) plays a role in the strength of the finding. In a real life example, National Science Foundation (NSF) conducted a study of bachelor's degree graduates with a science or engineering degree in 1977 and 1978. NSF reported that women earned 77% of the average salary of men. However, when the data were recalculated by taking into consideration the lurking variable of job type, the average job salary was at least 92% that of men. By combining all science and engineering jobs, the lower life science salaries in which more women were employed confounded the results. This example stresses the importance of gathering the right information.

Residual Confounding

Several situations occur in which confounding may be important. The three examples below are known as residual confounding.

Confounding by Unmeasured Variables

This one is the easiest concept to understand, but can also be the most evasive. The study results may vary or change directions, if an unknown variable is added to the equation. If the researcher had thought to collect data on this variable, it would not be "unknown."

Case Study: Antioxidant Vitamin Intake and Cardiovascular Disease Risk

Observational studies have shown a protective effect of antioxidant vitamin intake and the risk of developing cardiovascular disease (CVD). In other words, those who take Vitamin E are less likely to have heart attacks. However, randomized clinical trials (RCT) have shown no effect. One theory as to why an observational study's result differs from the RCT's results is due to confounding by behavioral and social factors acting across the life course. For example, childhood social class may be an important confounder. In order for an observational study to deal with the confounder, it needs to be measured perfectly. Failure to measure these life course factors could be the reason for the different results between observational and RCT studies.

Confounding by Unexamined Variables

Similar to confounding by unmeasured variables, confounding by unexamined variables means that the researcher had obtained the data but did not include it in the analysis. For example, in the case of mortality risk and plasma ascorbic acid, physical activity is considered a confounder. In one published study, data was gathered on physical activity but these data were not included in the model. If physical activity is truly a confounder, then omitting the confounder may have a sizable effect on the risk estimates for the relation between ascorbic acid and mortality.

Confounding by Measurement Error

In this case, the variable has been measured but not well. Food intake is an area in which there is almost always measurement error. Several techniques have been used to try to obtain good data on food intake but all methods have been found to have measurement error. Examples of food intake methods include daily logs, food frequency questionnaires, and duplicate diet (you fix 2 plates of food and one plate goes into a collection bin that is given to the researcher for nutrient analysis).

In the antioxidant vitamin intake and cardiovascular disease risk example, measurement error, may be present. The intake quantity of antioxidant vitamins in the observational studies was derived from food frequency questionnaires. Accurate reporting of food intake is known to contain measurement error and therefore the reported results may be driven by confounding by measurement error.

Residual confounding is an important concept to keep in mind; however, it should not paralyze the researcher. Doing a thorough literature review is a sensible step in obtaining information on potential confounders so that this data may be collected and included in the statistical models.

Effect Modifier

Another type of variable that can influence the study findings is an effect modifier. When the degree of association between an exposure and the health outcome changes according to the value or level of a third variable, this is called an effect modifier. Sex is a common effect modifier. For example, a hypothetical risk of a disease is 40 per 10,000 for women and 10 per 10,000 for men. The degree of association between risk and exposure changes from 40 to 10 per 10,000 based on sex. Therefore, sex is considered an effect modifier in this case.

One of the most familiar effect modifiers that has had significant public policy is alcohol consumption and driving. Driving is a risk factor for injury. Alcohol consumption is a risk factor for injury. However, drunk driving significantly increases the risk of injury.

It is an effect modifier.

Unlike confounding, in which the determination of a confounder is based on scientific reasoning, an effect modifier can be assessed statistically. One useful method to evaluate the possibility of an effect modifier is to stratify the data. For example, in a hypothetical study it was shown that roofers had a two fold increased risk of knee disorders than other types of construction workers, such as electricians or painters. However, when these two groups (plumbers and other construction workers) were stratified by normal weight and overweight, the overweight category showed a three fold increased risk and the normal weight category showed a slight increased risk for plumbers. Weight was an effect modifier.

Summary

In observational studies, especially where the researcher does not have control over all the characteristics of the population under study, lurking factors can significantly influence the findings of a study. Therefore, it is imperative that the context be considered in a study. A thorough reading of the literature can help the researcher be aware of potential confounders. Sometimes, it is just common sense thinking and applying that knowledge.

Concept Reinforcement

1. What is one piece of information that the researcher should collect in any observational study of lung cancer?

2. Epidemiologists are very likely to say something is associated with a health outcome but rarely that something causes a health outcome. Why do epidemiologists shy away from statements of causality?

3. What is the commonality between an effect modifier and a confounder?

Chapter 35 - Types of Bias

Chapter Objectives

- Define selection bias
- Define recall bias
- Define misclassification bias
- Explain Berkson's bias
- Define ecological fallacy

In designing a study and collecting information about participants, there is always some degree of error. Nothing is ever perfect. If it is random error, in other words errors that occur by chance, then the researcher is not as concerned. However if there are error in the design of the sampling plan or in the data collection that is not merely chance, then the results of the study maybe invalid. Sometimes all the researcher can do is note the type of error in the discussion of the published paper and let the readers decide about the validity of the study results. In this chapter, we are going to describe several types of errors which are also known as bias.

Bias

Bias is a systemic error. There is no set formula for interpreting the bias of a study. However, a set of questions should always be asked when reading or hearing about study results.

- How were the participants selected? In other words, how representative is the target population with regard to the hypothesis.
- Are those that participated different from those that did not participate in important ways?
- How accurate was the exposure and outcome variables measures?

Selection Bias

Who is given the survey in the first place? For example, a researcher is interested in the determining the reasons (predictors) of knee injuries in adolescents (aged 14-18 years) in San Bernardino Valley, California. The researcher sends a survey to all high school male athletes since the researcher knows this is the most injury prone group. This sampling design has selection bias since the researcher did not ask females. It is not unreasonable to consider that females may have different experiences that predict knee injuries. Furthermore, the researcher did not ask students who were not athletes. For both males and females who had sustained a knee injury in this population (athletes and non-athletes), the researcher did not gather complete information about predictors. The researcher did gather information on one sub-group, male athletes.

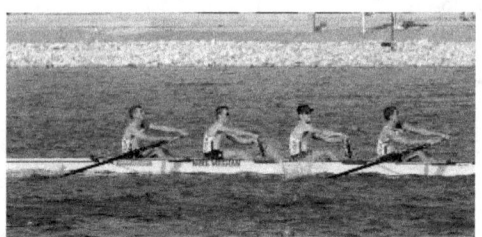

Referral Bias

If the population of sick people comes from one type of hospital, this may introduce referral bias. For example, in a famous study called the National Perinatal Collaborative Project (1959-1974) 12 prestigious hospitals participated in the project. The purpose of the project was to follow pregnant women and their babies for several years to determine risk factors associated with pregnancy and children's health. Many findings were reported but after several years, it was discovered that some of the health outcomes of the babies were much higher rates than the general population. This was because the hospitals that participated in the research were more likely to have women with high risk pregnancies as patients. This is an example of referral bias—high risk pregnant women were referred to these participating hospitals, not because of the research study but because they were considered the best hospitals in the region.

Interpretation Bias

If the question is not clearly written, respondents may answer the question differently than was intended. For example, "Is your work made more difficult because you have a child in daycare?"

A "no" response may mean, "No, I do not have a child in daycare" or "No, my work is not more difficult"

This interpretation bias can also occur in a medical setting. It is also called diagnostic bias. For example, if a radiologist is asked to look at a chest x-ray for signs of lung cancer and the radiologist knows the patient is a long time older heavy smoker, s/he may be more likely to examine the x-ray much more closely for any sign of cancer than for a young patient without a history of smoking. This behavior is good for clinical practice but is not good for research since it introduces bias. Participants are treated differently based on their smoking status.

Recall Bias

Asking participants about an event that happened long ago can create recall bias. For example, many people believe that someone with an illness often ask "why me?" It is common for patients to think back on their lives very carefully and remember details that they think might be associated with the disease. For example, it was found that mothers whose children have had leukemia were more likely than mothers of healthy children to remember details of diagnostic X-ray examinations during pregnancy.

Self-selection Bias

Another type of bias can occur if the participants volunteer for a study. This is known as self-selection bias. The question is whether the volunteers are the same or different in some important ways from a random sample of participants. A similar type of bias is when participants recommend their friends or relatives for the study. This is problematic from an analytical perspective since it is well known that friends and relatives are more similar than strangers. Again this violates the goal of a random sample of the population in which the results can be generalized to the population.

Interviewer Bias

No matter how professional an interviewer acts, there is always to possibility that the respondent is providing answers to the questions based on this relationship. For children this is readily apparent. Children will often say whatever the adult wants to hear. For adults this can take the form of pleasing the interviewer, avoiding answering an embarrassing question honestly, giving answers quickly and without thought to finish the interview, etc. All these permutations can influence the study findings since the "true" description of risk factors may not be accurately reflected in the participants' responses.

Berkson's Bias

Berkson's bias, also known as admission bias, was first described in 1946. The underlying concept is that people with more than one disease or condition are more likely to be hospitalized than people with just one disease or condition. Berkson's bias occurs when a researcher is exploring the relation between two diseases. An overestimation of exposed cases is likely to occur.

In addition to the study design and the data collection biases, there are also a couple of biases associated with screening.

Lead Time Bias

Even if someone is screened and found to have the disease, early detection does not prolong life. For example, clinical trials have shown that screening for lung cancer with chest x-ray will detect tumors in the lungs earlier; however the average survival time does not change with this earlier diagnosis. In other words, a person with lung cancer will live the same period of time with or without the screening test. The lead time bias can give the impression of the screening best being better since it prolongs life but in reality it just lets the patients know sooner about disease state.

Length Bias

For a slowly progressing disease, screening may find people with the disease at an earlier time. However, these slowly progressing diseases have better prognosis than quickly progressing diseases. In other words, patients with slowly progressing diseases will take longer to die from their disease. The mistaken idea is that the screened patients do better but this is a false perception. The screening identifies the disease earlier so there is a perceived increase in length of survival time. This increased length is just an artifice of the disease progression. In other words, the detection and treatment may not change the number of people diagnosed and the number of people who die from the disease every year.

Ecological Fallacy

It is important, when analyzing and interpreting data, to be precise in describing what the data tell you. Ecological fallacy is the result of an error of reasoning that occurs when the characteristics of a group of people are used to draw conclusions about an individual. Ecological fallacy occurs when people apply statistical information incorrectly. For example, a study of people who wear glasses shows that they have above-average intelligence. The ecological fallacy occurs when someone uses the information about the group to draw a conclusion about an individual who wears glasses. The person wearing the glasses may or may not have above-average intelligence.

Summary

A bias in the study design and data collection cannot be fixed. There is no analytical technique to correct for bias. Researchers spend considerable time thinking about the study design and data collection to minimize the different types of bias. Even with best efforts, if bias creeps into the study, the researcher will mention it in the discussion part of the published manuscript so the reader can decide about the validity of the study results.

Concept Reinforcement

1. What are some questions that you think your peers would be reluctant to give the "true" answer in a telephone interview? What could the interviewer say to encourage participants to answer "truthfully?"

2. Explain Berkson's Bias and its importance to health research.

3. How does length bias and lead time bias differ?

Chapter 36 - Generalizability

Chapter Objectives

- Discuss the importance of generalizability
- Define Type I error
- Define Type II error
- Describe the characteristics of participants in a study to increase generalizability

Generalizability

Generalizability is making predictions based on past, recurring experiences. We expect that the things that happen in the past will continue to happen in the future if the conditions remain the same. In epidemiology, researchers strive to collect generalizable data by using robust sampling techniques. These techniques are important to selecting a sample that is representative of the overall population. The results of the study are generalizable to the population only if the sample is representative of the overall population. Several situations can occur so that the study cannot be generalized.

Researchers use three types of generalizability. The first of these involves researchers determining if a specific treatment or intervention will produce the same results in different conditions. In this type of generalizability, the researchers need to determine whether some factor beyond the treatment generated the result they are studying. This helps establish the flexibility of the treatment, or its ability to adapt to new situations. The more flexible the treatment, the more adaptable it is to different situation.

A second form of generalizability focuses on measures rather than treatments. In this case, a result is generalizable if it produces the same results with different forms of measurement.

The third form of generalizability is related to the test subjects. The results of the test may be internally valid, meaning they are valid within the sample group, but not generalizable to the larger population because of differences between the test group and the overall population. In order for the results of a study to be generalizable, the sample group must reflect the characteristics of the larger population.

Characteristics of Populations

The populations of interest in epidemiologic studies have particular characteristics that are of interest to the researcher. Participants also have other characteristics that must be taken into account when designing the study and selecting the test group. There are general population characteristics, such as the racial and ethnic composition of the population, the percentage of men and women, the distribution of ages, socio-economic status, and marital status. There are also characteristics specific to the question the researchers asks, such as disease status, family history of disease, exposure history, etc.

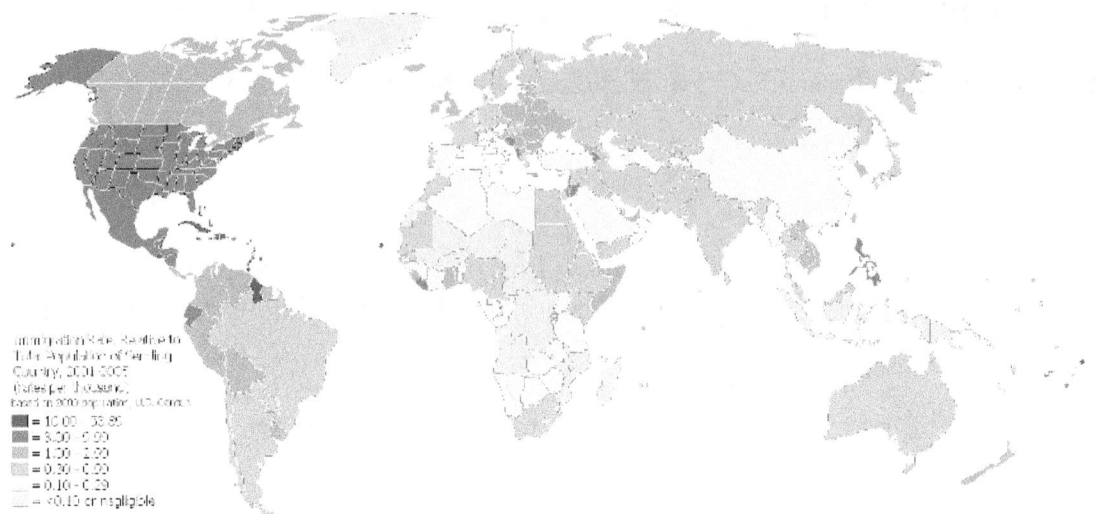

Shows the five-year (2001-2005) legal immigration rate per country's total 2000 population, defined as all those who received legal permanent residence in all categories, including regular immigrants, refugees and asylees, diversity lottery winners, NACARA/HRIFA beneficiaries, and others. This should be a good representation of the actual immigration rate, as the adjustment of status backlog was similar in size in 2000 and in 2005.

Immigrants from "Czechoslovakia (former)" included in data for Czech Republic, those from "Soviet Union (former)" included in data for Russia, and those from "Unknown country" conflated with Palestinian Territory. Corrections have been made for anomalous data for Congo (Brazzaville) vs. Congo (Kinshasa), Niger vs. Nigeria, and Guinea vs. Guinea-Bissau. Immigration from "Korea" equated with South Korea, with that from North Korea assumed to be negligible.

Think about whether the following study is generalizable. In this study, the larger population consists of high school graduates who decide to attend technical school. This population has the following characteristics: 18-21 years old, 75% male, 25% female. The researchers want to study why these people chose to attend technical school. The sample selected for the study consists of high school graduates ages 18-30 and is divided evenly between men and women.

Compared to the study population, all potential high school graduates range in age from 18-21 years old and are composed of 75% men and 25% women. The sample population has an age range of 18-30 years old and is divided evenly between men and women. The only thing that is consistent is that these two groups both consist of high school graduates.

The results obtained from the sample group will not be generalizable to the overall group because of the fundamental differences in the characteristics of the test group and the overall population. One means of figuring out if the makeup of the participants is similar to the overall population is to run a statistical test. If the differences are big enough, it is said to be statistically significant.

Error

All statistic tests contain some error. An important concept to understand when working in epidemiology is statistical error as it relates to significance testing. There are two basic types of error: Type I and Type II.

Type I error is essentially a false positive. The probability of a Type I error occurring is shown using the Greek letter alpha (α). It is called the Type I error rate.

Type II error is the opposite – a false negative. The Type II error rate, which is the probability of a Type II error, is shown using the Greek letter beta (β).

This concept can be shown using a 2x2 table. The columns indicate someone with a disease or without. The rows indicate someone with or without a risk factor.

	Disease, Illness, Injury	
	Positive	Negative
Risk Factor		
Positive	True	Type I Error
Negative	Type II Error	True

A 2x2 table includes four options.

- A person can have the disease and the risk factor. This is known as true positive. This means there are not any errors in the testing.

- A person does not have the disease and does not have the risk factor. This is known as a true negative. This means there are not any errors in the testing.

- A person does not have the disease but the test for the risk factor shows that the person has the risk factor. This is known as False positive. It indicates type I error.

- A person has the disease but the test for the risk factor shows that the person does not have the risk factor. This is known as False negative. It indicates type II error.

In any test, the magnitude of type I and type II errors vary. In the world of statistics and statistical testing there is always a balance between type I and type II errors. A large Type I error could result in a research reporting an association between a risk factor and a disease when one does not exist. In contrast a large Type II error could result in a researcher reporting no association between a risk factor and a disease when one really exists.

Summary

In order for epidemiologic studies to be generalizable, the sample group must reflect the larger population, both in composition and in terms of the specific question being asked. For example, if the question of interest is risk of cancer due to exposure to a certain chemical, the sample population must reflect the same characteristics as the overall population for cancer incidence and potential exposure. Epidemiologists face two specific types of error when studying populations. The first is Type I error, which is essentially a false positive. The second is Type II error, which is a false negative. In both cases the true situation is not represented.

Concept Reinforcement

1. Explain the importance of generalizability in epidemiologic studies

2. Describe the different between Type I and Type II error.

3. Explain how to improve generalizability by selecting the proper sample population.

Chapter 37 - Publication Bias

Chapter Objectives

- Describe publication bias and its implications
- Describe affiliation of author and its implication
- Describe implication of industry funded research and ownership of data

Having papers published is an important part of many researchers' jobs. The dissemination of research findings advances the field. However, publishing study results is not straightforward.

Publication Bias

Publication bias is the tendency, on average, for studies to be published in which the results are significant and for studies that did not find a significant finding to not be published. This tendency may result in scientists choosing to report only significant findings and not submitting manuscripts for publication in which the findings were not significant.

Steps Towards Publication

The researcher takes many steps to achieve a publication. The first step after a study is completed and the data are analyzed is to decide the journal that will receive their submission. Journals are informally ranked from top tier to fourth tier. The most prestigious journals are in the top tier. Having a paper published in a top tier journal carries much for prestige to the researcher and often is more widely read than a fourth tier journal.

After the researcher decides upon the journal, the manuscript is formatted to match the requirements of the journal. There are often word limits for the manuscript and details regarding the layout of the manuscript.

The manuscript is submitted to the journal and the editors look it over. This is the first place where publication bias can be felt. Editors may feel that non-significant findings are less likely to be interesting to their readership and therefore reject the manuscript. However, if the editors think it is interesting and it matches the journal's purpose, they then send it out for peer review.

A peer review process consists of two or three researchers reading the manuscript carefully and making comments and suggestion to improve it. The reviewers return the manuscript back to the journal editors and indicate whether the manuscript should be 1) accepted, no revisions, 2) accepted with minor revisions, 3) in need of major revisions or 4) rejected. Most manuscripts are given category 3 or 4 status. It is extremely rare to have a manuscript accepted without some changes suggested. This is the second point in the publication process where a manuscript with a non-significant finding may be rejected.

After the peer review process, the authors of the original manuscript have the opportunity to revise and resubmit their draft or try another journal with their manuscript.

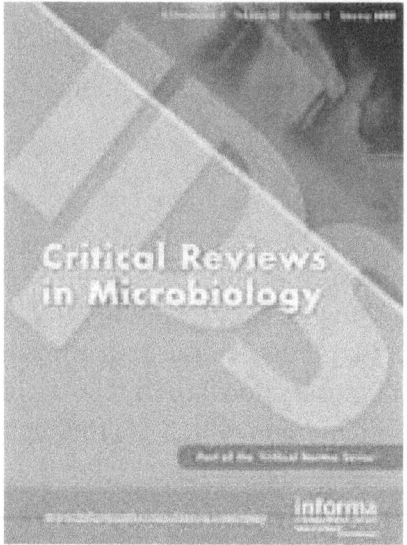

A manuscript is not published in respected scientific journals without the author disclosing a conflict of interests and stating their affiliation. The affiliation means the place where the authors work. A conflict of interest means that the author must disclose any money received from an institution or business that directly relates to the study. For example, if the researcher is studying the efficacy of a drug manufactured by a pharmaceutical company and the same pharmaceutical company gives the author a consulting fee, this would be disclosed on a conflict of interest statement.

Industry Funded-Research

In many cases, private companies (industry) sponsor research at independent research institutions or universities. The purpose of this research is usually to answer a specific question about a product or service provided by the company. The company who sponsors the research provides the funding for the research and helps define the research question being asked by the study. The researcher should independently perform the research and analyze the data to answer the question that was posed. Sometimes there are concerns about the influence of the company on the results of the study. There have been cases where the company has coerced the researcher into either designing the study to ensure a favorable result for the company or trying to quash unfavorable results. These cases have resulted in skepticism regarding the results of industry-sponsored research because of concerns about bias.

Sir Richard Doll

Sir Richard Doll is a famous epidemiologist. He, along with Ernst Wynder, Bradford Hill, and Evarts Graham, showed that smoking was linked to lung cancer and increased the risk of heart disease in the 1950s. He also studied asbestos and lung cancer, radiation and leukemia and alcohol consumption and breast cancer.

After his death in 2005, it was discovered that he had received consultancy payments for chemical companies whose products he defended in court. He received many payments. For example, one payment was for $1500 *per day* from Monsanto, a chemical company, which began in 1976 and continued to 2002. Most of these payments were never disclosed to the public. Sir Richard Doll has his defenders and those who feel his work is tainted since he did not disclose his conflict of interest.

Ownership of Data

Ownership of data is a critical issue in scientific studies. Universities tend to be very open in terms of the dissemination of research results. University faculty members are encouraged to publish their research results and report them at scientific meetings. In fact, the publication record of a faculty member is a key measure of success and performance. Many times, however, industry-sponsored research results in the company owning the research results. This can lead to suppression of the results for reasons of confidentiality or if they are not favorable to the company. In other situations, it can lead to inventions made during the course of the study not being further studied or commercialized.

Summary

Dissemination of study results to the wider audience of the research audience is critical for advancement of science. However, researchers depend on companies who are businesses to publish their findings, often for a nominal fee. The company relies on subscriptions to their journals to offset the costs of production. Editors may feel it is necessary to accept findings that are significant rather than non-significant findings to keep the readership numbers high, thereby leading to publication bias. One recent response to this well-known dilemma is that a few journals have added a section specifically for non-significant findings. Because research is expensive, great care has to be taken by the researchers to make sure their findings are not the result of a conflict of interest.

Concept Reinforcement

1. Do you think there is any problem with a researcher being paid as a consultant by a company in which the researcher is evaluating a device the company makes?

2. Can you think of any way in which pharmaceutical companies can get research done on their drugs without having any conflict of interest situations?

3. What do you think about Sir Richard Dolls' situation?

Chapter 38 - Crude Rate, Numerator and Denominator

Chapter Objectives

- Calculate crude rate
- Identify numerator and denominator
- Identify the proper denominator for a particular study

Once the data have been collected, the researcher publishes results in peer-reviewed scientific journals. There are several standard means to report results. The crude rate of a disease is one of those.

Crude Rate

A crude rate applies to the participants in the study without consideration of any characteristics of the participants. As the name implies the crude rate is generally the first impression of the results. Using the crude rate to compare studies or compare data should be done with extreme caution since the characteristics of the populations may differ. One of the most common differences between places is the age structure. In other words the percent of young, middle aged, and older people. Sometimes, the percent of males and females is very different by place. The crude rate does not take any of these differences into consideration.

Crude rates are used 1) when number of deaths/diseases is not known for the subgroups of the population. In other words, the overall death count is known but not the number of deaths by age groups; 2) the population size of the subgroups is unknown. In other words, the overall population under study is known but not the number of people in each age group; 3) when the number of people dead/diseased is too small. If the numbers are small, the statistics are not very reliable since a few additional deaths can change the rates by quite a bit.

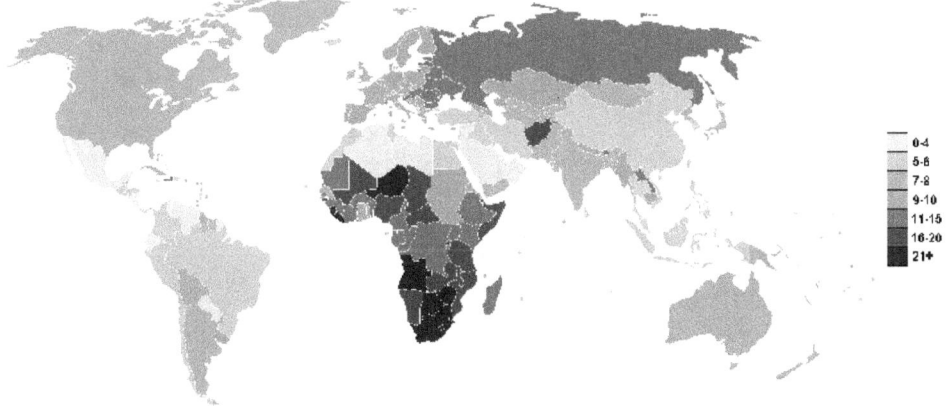

Crude mortality rate by country. The crude death rate for the world is about 8.23 per 1000 people.

Calculation of Crude Mortality Rate

Crude mortality rate (in a specified year) formula is number of deaths in the specified year ÷ mid year population (in the specified year) x 1000

Three pieces of information are needed to calculate the mortality rate:

A Defined Period of Time

It is necessary to have a defined population, with an estimate of the size of the population during the time period. Since people are always being born and dying, the population is never constant. Therefore, the population in any given year is the population at mid-year.

Count

The count is the number of deaths occurring over the designated period of time.

A Multiplier

The proportion can be multiplied by 1,000, 10,000 or 100,000, though is usually reported "per 1000." The reason to multiply by some number is that it is earlier to understand number of deaths as a whole number instead of a fraction. For example, a 0.0081 crude mortality rate is less understandable than 8.1 deaths per 1000 people.

Crude Mortality Rate Examples

Kuwait, United States, and Japan

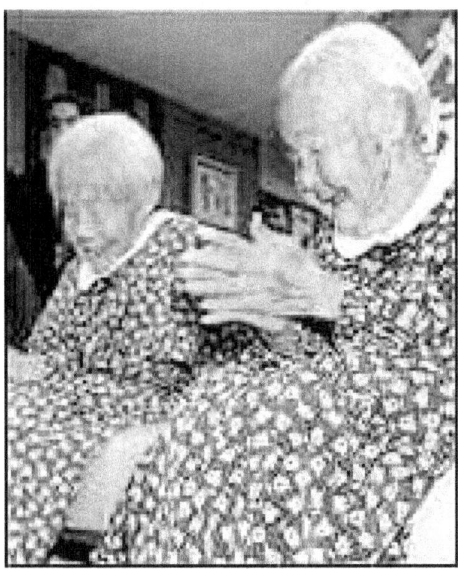

Oldest twins in modern history, Narita sisters, died at age 107

In the table below, Kuwait has the lowest crude mortality rate, substantially lower than the other countries listed, yet it also has the shortest life expectancy. This is an example in which the crude rate only provides a partial picture. By looking at the age distribution of the countries, you can see that Kuwait has substantially fewer people living to old age and a considerable number of children dying, compared to the other listed counties.

Crude mortality rate, life expectancy and age structure of selected counties, 2007 estimates					
			Percent population by age group		
Countries	Crude death rate	Life expectancy	0-14 yrs	15-64 yrs	65+ yrs
Kuwait	2.4	77.4	27%	70%	3%
United States	8.26	78.0	20%	67%	13%
Japan	8.98	83.5	14%	65%	21%
United Kingdom	10.09	78.7	17%	67%	16%

Example: The Difference Between Crude Rates in 2 Hypothetical Towns

In Northville, population of 100,000, 400 people died in 2008.

In Southville, population of 100,000, 700 people died in 2008.

The crude mortality rate is 4 per 1,000 in Northville and 7 per 1,000 in Southville, so these data tell us that Southville has a higher mortality rate. However, is there more to this story?

Age structure and mortality counts in Northville and Southville, population of each 100,000		
Age groups (in years)	Northville number of deaths	Southville number of deaths
<20	154	30
20-39	120	28
40-49	55	33
50-59	20	68
60-69	14	126
70-79	12	212
80-89	10	108
≥90	15	95
Total	400	700

Let's look at the age structure of the towns with the death counts, in the table. What does this table tell you? For some reason young people in Northville were more likely to die than those in Southville. In this situation, the story about death would focus on the reasons the young are dying in Northville because we all expect death to be a more common occurrence as we age.

Numerator and Denominator

When doing population studies, it is important to understand the relationship between the sample population and the entire population of interest. The relationships are often shown using fractions, which consist of numerators and denominators. The numerator is the sample population and the denominator is the overall population.

$$\frac{\text{Sample Population}}{\text{Total Population}}$$

Identifying the Proper Denominator

It is very important to find the proper denominator when designing, performing and analyzing the results of an epidemiologic study. The first step is to define the question the study will ask. Once that has been decided, the proper study population can be defined. If your question relates to the effects of pesticide exposure to farmer health, your study population (denominator) will be farmers. You will need to include farmers that use pesticides and farmers that do not use pesticides if you want to do a comparison. If you simply want to study the incidence of disease in farmers who use pesticides, you can include only those farmers who use pesticides.

Summary

Epidemiologists use many statistics to describe their study results. One type of result is a crude rate. This rate does not take into consideration any characteristics of the populations. It just shows the number or count of people with the disease, illness or heath outcome of interest in the numerator and the population at risk at midyear in the denominator. Crude rates have limited usefulness if other characteristics of the study population are important. When presenting data, epidemiologists take care in figuring out the denominator. They ask themselves, "Who makes up the population at risk?"

Concept Reinforcement

1. Explain crude rate and how to calculate it.

2. Describe how epidemiologic data are represented in a fraction.

3. Explain how to identify the proper denominator for an epidemiologic study.

Chapter 39 - Direct Standardization

Chapter Objectives

- Describe direct standardization
- Write the formula for calculating direct standardization
- Describe the situation in which this calculation is used

Standardized Rates

Although crude rates sometimes need to be used, the accepted practice is to standardize (also known as adjusted) the rates. Typically, the adjustment is based on age or some other population characteristic such as race or gender. Once this has been calculated, comparing rates makes more sense. With that said, it is also very important to look at the specific rates for any interesting differences or changes. In other words, our hypothetical towns of Northville and Southville would show some interesting specific age group rate differences that would not be apparent when looking at the overall mortality rate. A standardized rate differs from the crude rate in that the influence of some extraneous variable, typically age, has been removed.

Age structure and mortality counts in Northville and Southville		
Age groups (in years)	Northville number of deaths	Southville number of deaths
<20	154	30
20-39	120	28
40-49	55	33
50-59	20	68
60-69	14	126
70-79	12	212
80-89	10	108
≥90	15	95
Total	400	700

Two methods are commonly used to standardize the mortality rates, the direct method and the indirect method. In these two methods, standardization is just done by obtaining a weighted average. An example that students experience using weighted average is their class grade. This grade is almost always based on weights. For example, at the beginning of the year, the teacher tells the students that quizzes are worth 30%, homework are worth 20%, exams are worth 30% and final exam is worth 20%. The final class grade is computed using weighted averages: (0.3 times "averaged quiz grade") + (0.2 times "averaged homework grade") + (0.3 times "averaged exam score") + (0.2 times "final exam grade").

The first of two steps in standardization involves categorizing the populations under study into groups (also known as stratums (aka: strata)) based on some characteristic, such as age groups. The second step is calculating the stratum-specific rates. The third step is using a reference population. For example, if we are interested in comparing all cause mortality rates in two states, we will use the mortality rate by age groups from these two states. These rates would be standardized to a second population—often data from the US census. It can be state, national or world population rates. If the researcher is doing an age standardization (probably the most common standardization), then population proportions by age groups is used as the reference population.

Direct Standardization

In the direct method, a single population is used to standardize (weight) the rates for all comparisons. This is done by taking the sum of the products of stratum-specific mortality rates in the specific population being standardized and the stratum specific proportions of those strata in a standard population. Using the data below, multiply each stratum specific mortality rates in Florida by the US population proportion for each stratum, and then add these numbers for the mortality rate of each state.

$(6.96 * 0.01) + (0.33 * 0.05) + (0.15 * 0.07)....+ (129.05 * 0.02) = 7.5$ per 1000 for Florida

$(5.25 * 0.01) + (0.25 * 0.05) + (0.13 * 0.07)....+ (126.17 * 0.02) = 7.0$ per 1000 for California

If the direct standardization rate and the crude rate do not differ, this tells the researcher that the stratum specific variable (in this case age) was not different between the two populations. It is important to calculate both the crude and the standardization rates for this reason.

> **Crude rate**
>
> Remember the crude rate does not take into consideration any characteristic of the population, such as age structure. Therefore for Florida the crude mortality rate would be 168961/17384430 = 9.7 per 1000 people and for California the crude mortality rate is 232468/35842038 = 6.5 per 1000 people

Data needed to calculate direct and indirect standardization all cause mortality rates for Florida and California (from CDC Wonder database)

Age category	Florida 2004 population	Florida 2004 death	Florida stratum specific mortality rate	California 2004 population	California 2004 death	California stratum specific mortality rate	United States 2000 population	United States 2000 deaths	United States proportion	United States stratum specific mortality rate
<1	220,837	1,537	6.96	535,891	2,811	5.25	3,805,648	28,036	0.01	7.37
1-4	869,278	287	0.33	2,090,020	524	0.25	15,370,150	4,979	0.05	0.32
5-9	1,061,594	104	0.15	2,580,708	328	0.13	20,549,505	3,253	0.07	0.16
10-14	1,160,092	228	0.20	2,800,214	427	0.15	20,528,072	4,160	0.07	0.20
15-19	1,133,187	765	0.68	2,581,446	1,520	0.59	20,219,890	13,563	0.07	0.67
20-24	1,101,551	1,241	1.13	2,580,843	2,149	0.83	18,964,001	17,744	0.07	0.94
25-34	2,137,185	2,612	1.22	5,247,205	4,377	0.83	39,891,724	40,451	0.14	1.01
35-44	2,524,789	5,818	2.30	5,535,516	8,883	1.60	45,148,527	89,798	0.16	1.99
45-54	2,375,095	11,701	4.93	4,855,917	18,408	3.79	37,677,952	160,341	0.13	4.26
55-64	1,861,432	17,524	9.41	3,222,025	25,459	7.90	24,274,684	240,846	0.09	9.92
65-74	1,482,387	28,269	19.07	1,944,078	36,922	18.99	18,390,986	441,209	0.07	23.99
75-84	1,076,800	49,751	46.20	1,353,517	65,726	48.56	12,361,180	700,445	0.04	56.66
>84	380,203	49,064	129.05	514,658	64,934	126.17	4,239,587	648,171	0.02	152.89
total	17,384,430	168,961		35,842,038	232,468		281,421,906	2,392,995		

When the crude rate is higher than the directly standardized (age-adjusted) rates, this means that the age structure of the state is more unfavorable compared to the standardized population (e.g., United States age structure). In developed countries without the experience of infectious disease epidemics or war related deaths, age is one of the best predictors of death. Therefore, in this case, we would expect a higher proportion of people to die who are older and can conclude that the place with a higher crude rate reflects an older population.

To generalize these findings, we can say that if the direct age adjustment (direct standardization using age) produces a lower mortality rate, than the population of interest has a more *unfavorable* age distribution than the population that was used as the standard. In contrast, if the direct age adjustment produces a higher mortality rate, than the population of interest has a more *favorable* age distribution than the population that was used as the standard.

Summary

Direct standardization is one means of presenting study results so that other study results, that are also standardized in the same way can be compared to each other. To be able to directly standardize, data by stratum has to be available. If the crude rate and the direct standardization rates do not differ, this tells the researcher that the stratum specific variable is similar between the comparison groups. Although one number is the reported rate, it is also important to look at the age specific rates to identify any interesting patterns.

Concept Reinforcement

1. In which situation is it important to standardize rates?

2. Is there any situation in which crude rates are just as good as standardized rates?

3. What information is required to standardize rates?

Chapter 40 - Indirect Standardization

Chapter Objectives

- Describe indirect standardization

- Write the formula for calculating indirect standardization

- Describe the situation in which this calculation is used

In comparing the incidence or mortality rates between different places, it is rare that the characteristics of the two places are similar. If the important characteristics of two places such as the age structure, are similar, then a crude rate works just fine. However, if the characteristics are different or suspected to be different, then the rates need to be standardized so they can be compared to each other.

Standardized Rates

The accepted practice in epidemiology is to standardize (also known as adjust) the rates. The direct and indirect methods of standardization are the two most commonly used techniques for standardizing data. Using either of these methods, standardization is just obtaining a weighted average. An example that students experience using weighted average is their class grade. This grade is almost always based on weights. For example, at the beginning of the year, the teacher tells the students that quizzes are worth 30%, homework are worth 20%, exams are worth 30% and final exam is worth 20%. The final class grade is computed using weighted averages: (0.3 times "averaged quiz grade") + (0.2 times "averaged homework grade") + (0.3 times "averaged exam score") + (0.2 times "final exam grade").

Indirect Standardization

The indirect method is a little more complicated than direct standardization. It is used when stratum-specific rates are unavailable in the population of interest. It is also used when the number of deaths (or counts of disease) per stratum is small, say less than 5 or 10. Finally, the indirect method is used in occupational studies: studies that compare the death rate in an industry to the general population death rate. The question that the researcher asks is whether working in a particular occupation is more hazardous or not. Using these statistics, studies are produced which rank the most hazardous occupations.

The U.S. Bureau of Labor Statistics calculated the most hazardous jobs in 1994. Below are the top 20 most hazardous jobs.

Occupation	Relative Risk	Leading Fatal Event
Average All Jobs	1.0	Homicide and Accidents
Fishers	21.3	Drowning
Timber Cutters	20.6	Struck by object
Airplane Pilots	19.9	Airplane crashes
Structural Metal Workers	13.1	Falls
Taxi Cab Drivers	9.5	Homicide
Construction Workers	8.1	Vehicular, Falls
Roofers	5.9	Falls
Electric Power Installers/Repairers	5.7	Electrocution
Truck Driver	5.3	Highway Crashes
Farm Occupations	5.1	Vehicular
Police, Detectives, Supervisors	3.4	Homicide, Highway Crashes
Non-construction Laborers	3.2	Vehicular
Electricians	3.2	Electrocution
Welders and Cutters	2.4	Falls, Fires
Guards	2.3	Homicide
Ground Keepers and Gardeners	1.9	Vehicular
Carpenters	1.6	Falls
Auto Mechanics	1.1	Highway Crashes, Homicide
Supervisors, Proprietors, Sales	1.0	Homicide
Cashiers	0.9	Homicide

Calculation of Indirect Standardization

In the indirect method, two steps are used to calculate the rate. For simplicity, we will calculate a state's mortality rate using indirect standardization. Incidence rate can be used in the same way.

Data needed to calculate direct and indirect standardization all cause mortality rates for Florida and California (from CDC Wonder database)

Age category	Florida 2004 population	Florida 2004 death	stratum specific mortality rate	California 2004 population	California 2004 death	stratum specific mortality rate	United States 2000 population	United States 2000 deaths	proportion	stratum specific mortality rate
<1	220,837	1,537	6.96	535,891	2,811	5.25	3,805,648	28,035	0.01	7.37
1-4	869,278	287	0.33	2,090,020	524	0.25	15,370,150	4,979	0.05	0.32
5-9	1,061,594	164	0.15	2,580,708	328	0.13	20,549,505	3,253	0.07	0.16
10-14	1,160,092	228	0.20	2,800,214	427	0.15	20,528,072	4,160	0.07	0.20
15-19	1,133,187	765	0.68	2,581,446	1,520	0.59	20,219,890	13,563	0.07	0.67
20-24	1,101,551	1,241	1.13	2,580,843	2,149	0.83	18,964,001	17,744	0.07	0.94
25-34	2,137,185	2,612	1.22	5,247,205	4,377	0.83	39,891,724	40,451	0.14	1.01
35-44	2,524,789	5,818	2.30	5,535,516	8,883	1.60	45,148,527	89,798	0.16	1.99
45-54	2,375,095	11,701	4.93	4,855,917	18,408	3.79	37,677,952	160,341	0.13	4.26
55-64	1,861,432	17,524	9.41	3,222,025	25,459	7.90	24,274,684	240,040	0.09	9.92
65-74	1,482,387	28,269	19.07	1,944,078	36,922	18.99	18,390,986	441,209	0.07	23.99
75-84	1,076,800	49,751	46.20	1,353,517	65,726	48.56	12,361,180	700,445	0.04	56.66
>84	380,203	49,064	129.05	514,658	64,934	126.17	4,239,587	648,171	0.02	152.89
total	17,384,430	168,961		35,842,038	232,468		281,421,906	2,392,995		

First, the sum of the product of stratum-specific rates in the standard population and the proportion representation of those strata in the population being standardized is used to produce expected deaths. Then, the actual deaths in the population being standardized are divided by the expected deaths to produce standard mortality rates (SMR). SMR = actual deaths divided by expected deaths.

To determine the expected number of deaths, multiply the population of the state by the stratum specific mortality rate and divide by 1000, since the above stratum specific rates are per 1,000 and we want the expected total number of deaths.

((220,837 x 7.37) + (869,278 x 0.32) + (1,061,594 x 0.16)....+ (380,203 x 152.89))/1,000 = 194,575

Divide the state's actual number by the expected number (168,961 / 194,575) and then multiply by 100 = 87%. This is known as the standard mortality ratio (SMR). This means that deaths in Florida are 87% of the United States rates and for California they are 119% of the United States rates.

To review, the direct standardization gives an *expected rate* (standardized rate). This can be compared to the crude rate. An indirect standardization gives an *expected number of deaths*. This can be compared to the actual number of deaths in another population.

Summary

Public health researchers often used surveillance data routinely collected by governmental agencies, such as death certificates with underlying cause of death. As well as surveillance data, most governments undertake a census periodically, thus allowing researchers to apply methods discussed in this chapter to understand some trends in the health of a population.

Concept Reinforcement

1. Why is indirect standardization used instead of direct standardization method?

2. If the characteristics of two places are similar, does an epidemiologist need to standardize the rates? Explain

3. What is compared between populations in which indirect standardization is used?

Chapter 41 - Relative Risk

Chapter Objectives

- Construct a two by two table

- Write the formula for determining relative risk

- Explain the meaning of the point estimate

Epidemiologist use statistics to report study results. For certain study designs, one statistic that is commonly used is called relative risk. Cohort and randomized controlled trial studies report relative risk. Relative risk is defined as the ratio of the risk of disease or death among the exposed, to the risk among the unexposed.

Relative Risk

The relative risk can be measured by dividing the incidence rate in the exposed group by the incidence rate in the unexposed group. The value calculated is called a point estimate. A point estimate gives a single value along a scale. If the relative risk is 1.0, the risk of the outcome of interest is exactly equal for both the exposed and the unexposed groups. Therefore, the exposure did not have any effect on the health outcome. The further the relative risk is from 1.0, the greater the magnitude of effect. For example, a relative risk of 2.0 means that there is a two-fold increased risk for the health outcome in the exposed group compared to the unexposed group. Less than 1.0 implies a decrease risk. For example, a relative risk of 0.5 means the exposed group is 50% less likely to have the disease as the unexposed group. Another way to say increased or decreased risk is that an effect observed by a point estimate of less than 1.0 would be phrased as "less likely" and an effect observed by a point estimate of greater than 1.0 would be phrased as "more likely."

In epidemiology, it is not very useful to calculate a point estimate without also calculating a confidence interval. The formula for this calculation is beyond the scope to this lesson; however, interpretation of a confidence interval is within the scope of this lesson. If the confidence interval includes 1.0, there is no statistical difference between the intervention and control group. For example a point estimate of 1.3 with a 95% confidence interval of 0.8 – 1.5 means that there is no statistically significant increased risk. Similarly, if the point estimate is 0.6 and the confidence interval is 0.4 – 1.2, this also means there is not a decreased risk for the exposed group because 1.0 in within the confidence interval. In contrast, if 1.0 is not included in the confidence interval, the difference between the exposed and unexposed group would be considered statistically significant. If the point estimate is greater than 1.0, then the exposed group would be at a statistically significant increased risk and if the point estimate was less than 1.0, then the exposed group would be at a statistically significant decreased risk compared to the unexposed group.

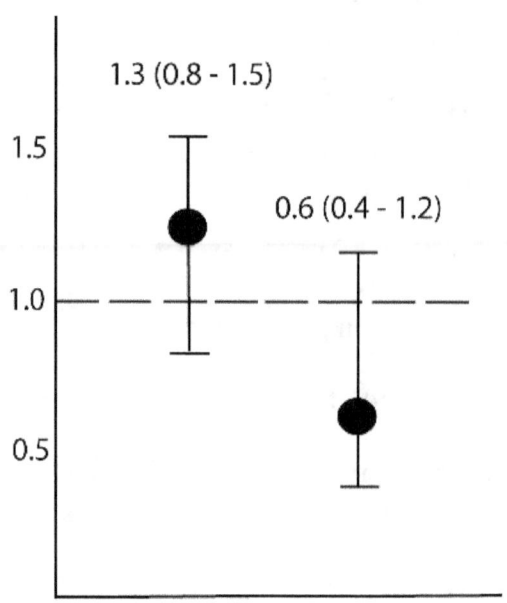

2 point estimates and 95% confidence intervals

Analysis of Study Data: Use of Two by Two Table

One important tool used to evaluate the association between exposure and disease is a two by two table. This is used in many calculations.

		Disease Status		
		Present	Absent	Total
Exposure Status	Present	A (exposure, disease present)	B (exposure, but no disease)	A + B
	Absent	C (no exposure, disease present)	D (no exposure, no disease)	C + D
	Total	A + C (total number with disease)	B + D (total number without disease)	N (sample total)

The columns represent disease status (with or without the disease) and the rows represent exposure status (present or absence of exposure). The convention for two by two tables should be constructed so that the first row should refer to those with the exposure of interest and the first column should refer to those with the disease.

This type of table cross-classifies exposure status and disease status. The total number of participants with the disease is A + C and the total number without the disease is B + D. In addition, the total number with exposure is A + B and those without exposure is C + D. The entry in cell A refers to those with the exposure and the disease present. The cell B refers to those with exposure but no disease. Cell C refers to those who were not exposed but have the disease. And finally cell D refers to those without the exposure and without the disease.

Order to Filling in the 2x2 Table by Study Type

In a cohort study design, the total number of study participants who have the exposure (A + B) and who do not have the exposure (C + D) is filled in first. In a cohort study design, the participants are followed over time. Cells (A, B, C, D) are filled in at the conclusion of the study or when the disease status is determined at some point during the study.

In a case control study design, the total number of study participants who have the disease (A + C) and without the disease (B + D) is filled in first. At the conclusion of the study, the exposure status (A, B, C, D) is filled in.

In the cross-sectional study design, enrolling a sample of participants (N) would be determined first. Next each participant's exposure and disease status would be identified (A, B, C, D). The totals (A + B) and (C + D) would be calculated last.

Calculation of Relative Risk

Relative risk is calculated with the following formula:

$$\text{Relative Risk} = \frac{\frac{A}{A+B}}{\frac{C}{C+D}}$$

This formula shows a ratio of the exposed to the unexposed. This is the essence of a relative risk calculation.

Summary

One statistic used by epidemiologist to describe study results is relative risk. This is a relative measure since it compares the exposed group to the unexposed group. Filling out a 2x2 table is helpful in understanding the calculation. If there is no difference between the two groups, the point estimate is 1.0. Only statistically significant differences between the exposed and unexposed group will have a confidence interval that does not contain one.

Examples of point estimates and confidence intervals, statistical significance			
Point estimate	**Confidence Interval**	**Includes 1.0**	**Statistically significant**
1.75	1.2 – 2.3	No	Yes
2.80	2.3 – 4.9	No	Yes
1.22	0.8 – 1.4	Yes	No
0.76	0.2 – 0.9	No	Yes
0.37	0.3 – 0.5	Yes	Yes
0.94	0.7 – 1.6	No	No

Concept Reinforcement

1. What is the purpose of a two by two table?

2. Why do fields need to be filled in in different order depending on study type?

3. What is important about statistically significant findings?

Chapter 42 - Odds Ratio

Chapter Objectives

- Construct a two by two table
- Write the formula for determining odds ratio
- Explain the meaning of the point estimate

For case control studies, odds ratio is the statistic used to explain the differences between exposed and unexposed groups. In other words, odds ratio is the ratio of the probability of occurrence of an event to the probability of the event not occurring.

Odds Ratio

The odds ratio measures the odds of exposure of a specified disease. Similar to relative risk, an odds ratio of 1.0 means that the odds of exposure is equal between cases and controls and that the risk factor is not associated with the disease. An odds ratio greater than 1.0 suggests an increase risk of the disease based on a particular exposure. In contrast an odds ratio less than 1.0 suggests a lower risk for the disease based on a particular exposure.

Odds ratios should be interpreted with caution. One reason is that a case-control study is retrospective by design with only one period of observation. Only prospective studies can determine rates and consequently risks. The reason that a case-control study cannot determine rates and true risks is based on the way in which the study groups are assembled. In a case-control study, the total number of participants who are exposed (A + B) and the total number of participants who are not exposed (C + D), do not represent the total population of exposed and non-exposed individuals. Consequently there is no appropriate denominator for the population at risk and therefore no way to directly determine disease rates. However, with that said, if three conditions are met, the odds ratio provides a good approximation of the relative risk.

- The controls are representative of the target population in the frequency of the exposure of interest
- The cases are representative of all cases with regard to severity and diagnostic criteria
- The frequency of the disease in the population is small.

In the exposed group, the odds of a disease (exposed with the disease divided by exposed without the disease) provides similar results as risk (exposed with the disease divided by total number exposed to the disease) of a disease when the proportion of study participants with the disease is small and those with and without the disease are from the same relevant population.

		Disease Status		
		Present	Absent	Total
Exposure Status	Present	A (exposure, disease present)	B (exposure, but no disease)	A + B
	Absent	C (no exposure, disease present)	D (no exposure, no disease)	C + D
	Total	A + C (total number with disease)	B + D (total number without disease)	N (sample total)

Odds Ratio Calculation

The formula for calculating the odds ratio is:

$$\text{Odds ratio} = \frac{\frac{A}{C}}{\frac{B}{D}} \overset{\text{Mathematically Simplified}}{=} \frac{AD}{BC}$$

Formula for odds ratio

The important point to remember is that in a well-designed case-control study, the odds ratio is a good estimate of the risk ratio that could have been obtained from a more costly and time consuming prospective cohort study.

The same interpretation applies for the odds ratio as it does for the relative risk. A point estimate gives a single value along a scale. If the odds ratio is 1.0, the odds of the outcome of interest is exactly equal for both the exposed and the unexposed groups. Therefore, the exposure did not have any effect on the health outcome. The further the odds ratio is from 1.0, the greater the magnitude of effect. For example, an odds ratio of 2.0 means that there is a two-fold increased risk for the health outcome in the exposed group compared to the unexposed group. Less than 1.0 implies a decrease risk. For example a odds ratio of 0.5 means the exposed group is 50% less likely to have the disease as the unexposed group.

Absolute Versus Relative Measure

Risk can be measured in two ways, as an absolute measure or as a relative measure.

Absolute Measure

Absolute risk provides the number at risk. It is an actual number. For example, as a simple example, if 10 women in a town of 10,000 adult women are diagnosed with cervical cancer, the absolute risk of cervical cancer in the town is 10 per 10,000. However, the people in the town have different lifestyles, genes, living conditions which absolute risk does not take into consideration.

With more calculations, the attributable risk can be calculated. Attributable risk means the number of people who get the diseased due to the exposure. On the flip side, it can also be used to indicate the number of people who would not get the disease if they were not exposed. Population attributive risk tells us how much of the disease or health outcome can be attributed to a specific exposure in the total population. The population attributable risk is useful for policy makers.

The population attributable risk depends on the magnitude of the relative risk and the prevalence of exposure in the population. In other words, if not very many people have the disease, then the population attributable risk will not be very high. In contrast, common exposure may account for a large attributable risk. If only 2 people chew betel nut in a rural city, population of 50,000, and 1000 people are diagnosed with lip cancer from this population, then the relative risk from chewing betel nuts will be small. Similarly, if only 2 people contract a rare lip disease from a population of 50,000, the prevalence would be very small. In both of these hypothetical cases the population attributable risk would be small. In contrast smoking cigarettes is common in men in China (~60%) and the risk of lung cancer is also high in smokers (95% of lung cancer occurs among smokers). Therefore, the population attributable risk of lung cancer from exposure to smoking for men in China would be quite high.

Relative Measure

Relative measures (such as odds ratio or relative risk) indicate how strongly an exposure is associated with a particular disease. The relative measure does not give an indication of the impact of the exposure associated with the incidence of the disease in the population. A large statistically significant point estimate does not translate into more people with the disease; it does mean that the likelihood of disease associated with the exposure is high.

Summary

In case-control studies, the common statistic to report study results is odds ratio. This is an estimate of relative risk. It is a measure of the odds of the exposure of a given disease. Both relative risk and odds ratio are examples of relative measures since they provide information on the magnitude of the risk of disease from the exposure. Absolute measures provide useful information for policy makers because these statistics indicate the number of people affected by the exposure.

Concept Reinforcement

1. What is the difference between relative risk and absolute risk?

2. Why is prevalence important to know when calculating absolute risk?

3. Why is it possible to use odds ratio as an estimate of relative risk?

Chapter 43 - Confidence Interval

Chapter Objectives

- Define confidence interval

- Explain the relation between sample size and confidence interval

- Explain the use of 95% versus other percentages for CI

Sample Size Considerations

How big does a sample need to be? The bigger the sample size, the smaller the random error and the higher the likelihood of finding an effect. However, the bigger the sample size, the more expensive (and possibly more time consuming) the study. Researchers weigh these two competing interests: reduction of random error and resource allocation.

If a sample is too small in a probabilistic sample, the researcher will run into one of two problems. He/she may fail to find any meaningful result or not be able generalize the findings to the group or population.

If the sample size is too big, then:

1. there has been a waste of resources since the researcher need not have gathered all that data.

2. there has been a waste of respondents' time since some of their data were not needed.

3. a very large study has the power to find significant results for very small, even clinically inconsequential, differences.

When figuring out how many people to survey, the researcher realizes that as the population size increases, the percentage of people needed to achieve a high level of accuracy decrease rapidly. In other words, to obtain the same level of confidence in the study results, for larger population the researcher would need a smaller percentage of people surveyed and for a smaller population the researcher would need a larger percentage of people surveyed.

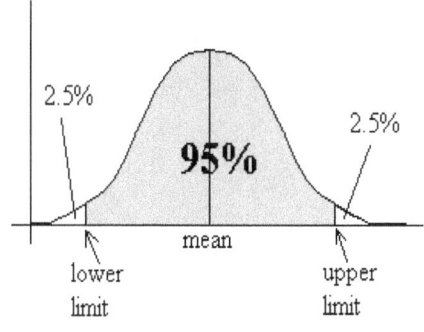

As noted above, all data have some error (variations). The technique to show the amount of variation in the data is to report the confidence interval. This means that in the distribution of data, the lower confidence interval point and upper confidence interval point in which 95 out of 100 samples of the specified size will be within the specified percent error of the study response. A rule of thumb is the larger the study size, the narrower the confidence interval. A second rule of thumb is the rule of diminishing return. This means that the researcher needs significantly more study participants to reduce the margin of error from 2 percent to 1 percent than from 5 percent to 4 percent. Just as a refresher, error is the amount of data variability around the reported result. Error can be shown as + and − value. For example if the researcher says men's ear's length at age 90 is 75.7 mm with 95% confidence interval of 71.2-80.2, that would mean that the error is ± 4.5 mm. The ear lengths could be as long as 80.2 or as short as 71.2, and in 100 studies 95 out of 100 studies, the men would have an ear length between 71.2 and 80.2.

95% Versus 99% Confidence Interval

There is not any reason that researchers use 95% CI instead of say 94% or 96%. It is just the convention. When a study reports 99% CI, this indicates that the researchers want to be very sure of their results. As a refresher, 99% CI means that in 100 studies, all but one study would find the same range of results. That is pretty impressive.

Example of 95% CI

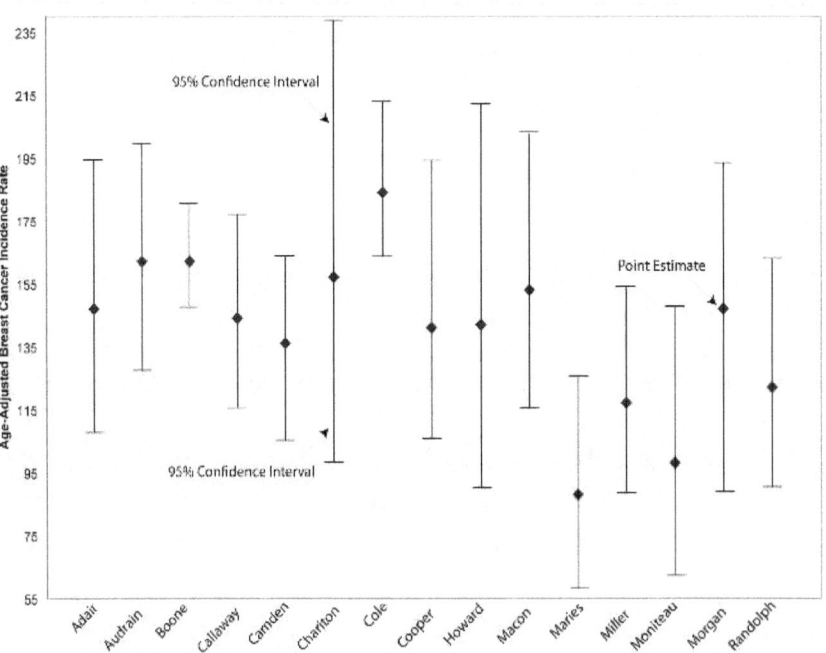

Age-adjusted breast cancer rates with 95% confidence intervals in 15 counties in Missouri

Using breast cancer data for 15 counties in mid-Missouri, the breast cancer rate varied from 184 per 100,000 people to 88 per 100,000 people. However, the confidence intervals for these counties mostly overlap each other. For example, Audrain and Boone counties have slightly different breast cancer rates. Boone County's confidence interval is completely within Audrain County's confidence interval. When confidence intervals overlap, this means that the results from overlapping confidence intervals are similar.

Summary

Confidence interval is an important concept when analyzing statistical data, including those generated by epidemiologic studies. Confidence interval is used to show the amount of variation in the data. The larger the study sample, the narrower the confidence interval of the study. Additionally, the rule of diminishing returns applies to reducing the confidence interval. It is easier to reduce the confidence interval from 5% to 4% than from 2% to 1%. Confidence intervals are typically stated in percentages with 95% confidence interval the most common. When confidence intervals overlap, this means that the results are similar.

Concept Reinforcement

1. Explain the concept of confidence interval.

2. Describe how sample size and confidence interval are related.

3. Discuss why 95% is used for confidence intervals.

Chapter 44 - Evidence-Based Research

Chapter Objectives

- Describe the characteristics of evidence-based research
- Describe the benefits of using evidence-based research
- Describe the 2010 Healthy People Program

Epidemiologists often have many ideas about what to study and what programs may be helpful. Historically, someone could make a suggestion and launch a program. However, these days to launch a program more and more funding agencies want the researcher to show that the program has a good chance of being successful. Funding agencies are requiring that the researcher show evidence of success. This can be evidence from a similar program, possibly with a different population or it can shown by using evidence from other research that explore the underlying characteristics of the population.

Evidence-based Research

Evidence-based research is research that builds on the results of prior research and takes advantage of existing research and knowledge to develop an effective plan for answering the question of interest.

Evidence-based research is beneficial because it guides researchers as they are developing new research programs. They are able to look at the results of previous research while developing new research studies.

Evidence-based research is becoming more and more popular as criteria for funding programs. It is also being used more and more in the medical field to determine the best practices for taking care of patients.

Healthy People 2010

Every 10 years the U.S. Department of Health and Human Services provides science-based national objectives for promoting health and preventing disease. Each state either adapts the Healthy People objectives or n   r states.

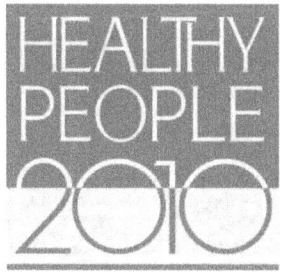

Healthy People 2010 is a list of specific health goals for the United States for which progress can be measured over time. In 1980, the first set of national health objectives was identified. At the beginning of each decade, the previous decade's health objectives are evaluated and new goals are set. Healthy People 2010 is the current set of health objectives for the nation. In 2009, meetings are being held to create the Healthy People 2020 objectives.

To create the Healthy People objectives, scientific studies over the previous 10 years are reviewed, new knowledge gained during the previous decade, trends in health, and technological innovations are incorporated into the new objectives.

Healthy People 2010 Goals

There are two broad goals of Healthy People 2010:

1. Improve quality of life and increase life expectancy
2. Eliminate health disparities

Disparity definition

The National Institute of Health defines disparities as the "differences in the incidence, prevalence, mortality, and burden of disease and other adverse health conditions that exist among specific population groups in the United States."

No "rule" exists to say at what point a difference between the overall average and the race/ethnic/specific population average indicates disparity. However, the Urban League of Pittsburgh suggested a 30% difference. This amount is more than would likely occur by chance.

The top health outcomes that have significant disparities—meaning differences in incidence, prevalence, and mortality-in order are cardiovascular disease, cancer, diabetes, HIV/AIDS, infant mortality, asthma, and mental health.

Healthy People 2010 Health Outcomes

For Healthy People 2010, 28 health outcomes have been identified to be measured and followed to determine improvement in the two broad goals. These health outcomes range from chronic diseases such as cancer to family planning to food safety.

- Access to Quality Health Services
- Arthritis, Osteoporosis, and Chronic Back Conditions
- Cancer
- Chronic Kidney Disease
- Diabetes
- Disability and Secondary Conditions
- Educational and Community-Based Programs

- Environmental Health
- Family Planning
- Food Safety
- Health Communication
- Heart Disease and Stroke
- HIV
- Immunization and Infectious Diseases
- Injury and Violence Prevention
- Maternal, Infant, and Child Health
- Medical Product Safety
- Mental Health and Mental Disorders
- Nutrition and Overweight
- Occupational Safety and Health
- Oral Health
- Physical Activity and Fitness
- Public Health Infrastructure
- Respiratory Diseases
- Sexually Transmitted Diseases
- Substance Abuse
- Tobacco Use
- Vision and Hearing

Within each of these health outcomes, specific objectives have been set. Overall, more than 450 objectives have been written.

Summary

With the improved technological capacity for rapid dissemination of scientific findings, evidence-based research is becoming a requirement by funding agencies. It is also becoming more important in medical care. Along with evidence-based research, is the use of a unifying framework towards improved public health is the Healthy People 2010 goals. It is updated every 10 years using evidence of the health of the population as well as innovations from the previous decade.

Concept Reinforcement

1. Explain evidence-based research.

2. State the benefits of evidence-based research.

3. Discuss the goals of the Healthy People 2010 program.

Chapter 45 - Public Policy

Chapter Objectives

- Define policy
- List five mechanisms used by government to implement policy change
- Describe Heberlein's three broad fixes to problems

Policy is a set of underlying principles that are used to guide programs at the municipal, state, national or international level. In this case, we are interested in policies that influence health promotion, protection, and services.

Many public policies are linked to health. Income support (assistance), environmental protection, housing support, and transportation policies are all examples of policies that can be linked to improved health of the population.

Mechanism for Implementing Policy

The list of how to implement a policy is quite long. Policy implementation may use several mechanisms simultaneously depending on the whether the policy is being considered on a larger scale, whether it is a newly enacted policy, who is responsible for the policy, etc.

One tool to implement a policy is establishing a policy as law. A classic public health policy is the required use of seat belts by drivers in most states. However, if a law is enacted and there is not any enforcement or regulation, the compliance may be less than perfect. Consequently, not only are some public health policies enacted as laws but they also have an enforcement component. For example, if a driver is seen without a seat belt, then in many states, the driver can be fined.

Sometimes public policy is supported through taxation. The Medicaid program is a federal program that supports many health programs. An example of one program supported by federal dollars, which are really our tax dollars, is the breast cancer and cervical screening program to women who cannot afford these tests. Another example is the WIC (Women, Infants, and Children) nutritional program. One part of this program is to provide prenatal care to pregnant women.

Three Strategies for Fixing a Societal Problem

Heberlein, a rural sociologist, wrote a paper in 1974 describing three strategies to fix a societal problem. He argued that the three ways to resolve any societal problem are through a technological fix, a cognitive fix or a structural fix. He used the example of intervening to reduce the pollution from 2-cycle boat engines on an inland lake. The technological fix is to design an engine that emits virtually no contaminants into the water. The cognitive fix is to educate the public on the pollution caused by 2-cycle motors and encourage their reduced use. The structural fix is removing the boat ramp so that boaters are unable to launch their motorized boats. This provocative idea can be applied to public health problems too. However, underlying these fixes is the need for money to implement them.

Delay Between Epidemiology Study Results and Policy Illustration

In a perfect world, policy should be based completely on evidence. However, this is rarely the case. Epidemiology studies are the source of the evidence considered when making policy. Consider the following classic epidemiology study.

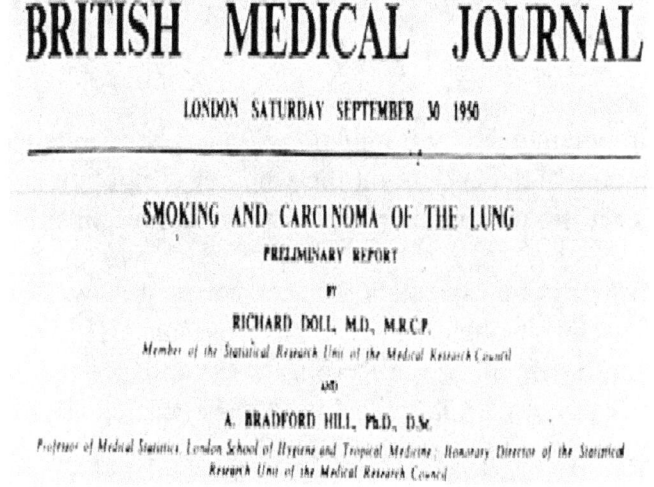

In 1950, Richard Doll and Bradford Hill published a study in the British Medical Journal that showed that smokers are at a 50 times greater risk for lung cancer.

By 1964, the Surgeon General announced to headline news that smoking was deleterious to one's health. This decision was based on reviewing more than 7,000 scientific articles, many of which were epidemiology studies.

By the beginning of the 21st century, places across the United States are banning smoking in public places such as restaurants, bars, and taverns. Lots of reasons can be cited as to why smoking is still common when unequivocal detrimental health effects are directly associated with smoking—both to the smoker, to the fetus, to the family exposed to second hand smoke. Both social pressure (i.e. to be "cool") and addiction contribute to people continuing to smoke. Further, the media and advertising efforts have also influenced continued use of tobacco. For example, movies are now featuring cigarette brands using close up shots and the number of actors smoking in movies has skyrocketed.

Precautionary Principle

The precautionary principle was formalized in Racine, Wisconsin at the 1998 Wingspread Conference. The following statements comprise the reasoning behind the precautionary principles as determined by the conference attendees. The key elements of the precautionary principle include taking precaution in the face of scientific uncertainty; exploring alternatives to possibly harmful actions; placing the burden of proof on proponents of an activity rather than on victims or potential victims of the activity; and using democratic processes to carry out and enforce the principle-including the public right to informed consent. Several aphorisms in the English language also support the precautionary principle. For example, "an ounce of prevention is worth a pound of cure" or a medical aphorism "first, do not harm."

Although this principle seems simple and reasonable, application of the principle has proven to be difficult. Critics of the precautionary principle say that it is impractical because the launching any new technology has inherent risks and potential for negative consequences. Additionally, the implementation of the precautionary principle would put additional economic burden on the proponents of the proposed activity.

Summary

The concept of public good is pervasive in health policies. Some polices target those in need. To participant in a federal or state sponsored program almost always is based on financial need. Most laws related to public health have the scales tipped towards the good of all whereas the rights of the individuals are considered less important. A once powerful concept, called the precautionary principle, argued that when in doubt about the harm that something might inflict on the population, a more conservative approach should be taken.

Concept Reinforcement

1. Of Heberlein's three fixes, which one do you think is most effective for public health issues and why?

2. What basic tenet of Americans is in conflict with the Precautionary Principle?

3. To what degree should your rights as a citizen be infringed upon for the good of all? For example, should you be required to get a vaccine to go to school? Is there a clear line between the rights of the individual versus the public good? Who should decide what is sufficient?

www.ingramcontent.com/pod-product-compliance
Lightning Source LLC
Chambersburg PA
CBHW062319220526
45469CB00008B/2568